A Patient's Guide to

Chinese Medicine

A Patient's Guide to
Chinese Medicine

Dr. Shen's Handbook of
Herbs and Acupuncture

Joel Harvey Schreck

Bay Tree Publishing
Point Richmond, California

Book design by mlTrees

Library of Congress Cataloging-in-Publication Data

Schreck, Joel Harvey.
  A patient's guide to Chinese medicine : Dr. Shen's handbook of herbs and acupuncture / by Joel Harvey Schreck.
    p. cm.
  Includes index.
  ISBN 978-0-9801758-0-6
  1. Medicine, Chinese--Popular works. 2. Herbs--Therapeutic use--Popular works. 3. Acupuncture--Popular works. I. Title.

R601.S37 2008
610--dc22
                          2008035301

Contents

Preface   Getting Started   viii

Acknowledgements and Confessions   xiv

Chapter 1   Methods of Chinese Medicine   1
                 Acupuncture
                 Moxibustion
                 Massage and Bodywork
                 Meditation, Movement, and Martial Arts
                 Herbal Medicine

Chapter 2   A Patient's Guide to Acupuncture and Herbs   8
                 What Patients Expect from Practitioners
                 Accreditation and Kinds of Practitioners
                 What Practitioners Expect from Patients
                 Stay the Course
                 Herbal Pointers
                 How to Take Pills
                 How to Drink Decoctions
                 How to Take Tinctures and Elixirs
                 How to Take Milled Powders and Granules
                 California Proposition 65 Warning Labels
                 Acupuncture Pointers
                 Chinese Medicine in the U.S. Health Care System

Chapter 3   Understanding Theories of Chinese Medicine   28
                 Qi and Blood
                 Yin and Yang
                 The Eight Principles
                 The Fourteen Channels
                 The Five Phases
                 The Five Emotions
                 The Twelve Organs
                 Applying the Theories

Chapter 4   Chinese Medicine in Action: Case Studies   41
Diagnosing Olga
Mr. Brown and Mr. Silver
John, Rita, and Patrick

Chapter 5   Famous Herbal Medicines   50
The Value of Combining Herbs
How Formulas Are Created
Famous Formulas

Chapter 6   Treatment of Ailments A to Z   71
Acne • Addictions: Alcohol, Nicotine, and Other Substances • Allergies •
Azheimer's • Arthritis, Bursitis, Tendonitis, and Joint Pain • Asthma • ADD,
ADHD, and Compulsive Behavior • Back Pain • Bleeding Disorders • Cancer •
High Cholesterol • Cold and Flu • Constipation • Cysts and Other Accumula-
tions • Depression and Anxiety • Diabetes • Digestive Problems • Ear Problems:
Ear Ringing and Hearing Loss • Eczema, Psoriasis, and Other Inflammatory
Skin Conditions • Energy Issues and Chronic Fatigue • Epilepsy and Seizures •
Hair Loss and Prematurely Gray Hair • Headaches • Heart Health • Hepatitis
• Hemorrhoids • High Blood Pressure (Hypertension) • Immunity • Infertility,
Pregnancy, and Miscarriage • Injury, Trauma, and Pain • Insomnia, Anxiety, and
Restlessness • Irritable Bowel Syndrome • Lice • Menopause and Hot Flashes •
Nausea, Vomiting, Gastric Reflux, and Morning Sickness • Pain • Prostate Con-
ditions • Sexual Problems • Thyroid Problems • Vaginal Yeast Infections • Warts •
Weight Gain, Weight Loss, and Diets • Zoster and Other Viruses

Chapter 7   Herbs and Their Categories   154
Introduction • Herbs That Release Exterior Conditions • Warm Pungent Herbs
for Releasing the Exterior • Cool Pungent Herbs for Releasing the Exterior •
Herbs That Clear Heat • Herbs That Clear Heat and Cool the Blood • Herbs
That Clear Heat and Dry Dampness • Herbs That Clear Heat and Clean Tox-
ins • Herbs That Clear and Relieve Summer Heat • Herbs That Drain Down-
ward • Purgatives • Moist Laxatives • Harsh Cathartics • Herbs That Drain
Dampness • Herbs That Expel Wind and Damp from the Surface • Herbs That
Transform Phlegm and Stop Coughing • Herbs to Transform Hot Phlegm •
Herbs to Transform Cold Phlegm • Herbs That Relieve Coughing and Wheez-
ing • Herbs That Transform Dampness • Herbs That Relieve Food Stagnation
• Herbs That Regulate the Qi • Herbs That Regulate the Blood • Herbs That

Nourish the Blood • Herbs That Vitalize the Blood • Herbs to Stop Bleeding • Herbs That Warm the Interior • Herbs That Strengthen (Tonifying Herbs) • Herbs That Tonify the Qi • Herbs That Tonify the Yang • Herbs That Tonify the Yin • Herbs That Astringe • Herbs That Nourish the Heart and Settle the Spirit • Herbs That Nourish the Heart • Herbs That Settle the Spirit • Aromatic Herbs That Open the Orifices • Herbs That Extinguish Interior Wind and Stop Tremors • Herbs That Expel Parasites • Herbs for Topical Application

Appendix 1: Chinese Herb List and Pronunciation Guide   196

How to Pronounce Chinese Words
List of Chinese Herbs

Appendix 2: The Organs: Their Functions, Correspondences, and Characteristics   208

The Five Viscera
The Six Bowels

Appendix 3: The Processing and Purity of Chinese Herbs   212

How Herbs Are Processed
Potential Impurities in Herbs
Western Drugs in Chinese Patent Medicines

Appendix 4: Food as Medicine   221

Appendix 5: Resources   224

Reading List
U.S. Schools of Chinese Medicine
Manufacturers of Chinese Medicine

Glossary   241

Index   246

Preface

Getting Started

Chinese medicine is the world's oldest, most comprehensive, original holistic medicine. It is practical, safe, reliable, and natural. Hundreds of modern, controlled studies have validated the effectiveness and safety of this ancient practice. This book introduces the ideas and treatments of Chinese medicine in a do-it-yourself reference guide for daily use.

I have practiced Chinese medicine near the University of California at Berkeley for over twenty-five years. When new clients show up at my clinic, they often say, "You are my last hope. I've tried everything." "Everything but Chinese medicine," I usually reply. Then I treat them, and they usually get better. And they are amazed. "Why didn't anyone tell me about this before?" they ask.

As a young man in 1970, I had not heard of Chinese medicine and never could have imagined using it, let alone practicing it. It took four separate "miracles" to turn me from a skeptic into a believer, and, finally, to the zealot I am today. Each of these eye-opening experiences peeled away a layer of doubt. In retrospect, I realized how clouded my vision had been before.

It began with my wife Betty's backache. Since adolescence, she had been enduring episodes of agonizing lower back pain. These attacks laid her out for days, sometimes weeks at a time. The worst attack occurred just after our first child was born, in 1971. Seeing Betty numbed on codeine and unable to nurse our newborn, a friend suggested that we try acupuncture, which, at the time, was illegal.

That first acupuncture treatment, performed in secret by an elderly Asian man in the back of a musty Chinatown storefront, was more than a novel experience. It was a revelation. Betty entered his office in pain and left it pain free. Though the problem returned, that first treatment made her willing to try again. Several years later, Betty underwent a series of acupuncture treatments. She has never since suffered from lower back pain.

My second wake-up call was my own first acupuncture treatment for excruciating neck pain. It was particularly hard for me, because I have always been squeamish around needles. Perhaps this is a strange admission for an acupuncturist, but as it turned out, I was rewarded for facing my fear. The acupuncturist seemed to grasp my dread instinctively, and stopped the neck pain by using a single needle in my wrist. I was astonished.

The third epiphany came when I brought a friend to see an acupuncturist for treatment of inflammatory bowel disease. My friend's prognosis was poor. The prescriptions caused terrible side effects, and radical surgery was deemed the ultimate "cure" for this condition. Alternatives seemed worth trying. When my friend didn't respond to acupuncture treatments, we tried Chinese herbal therapy. It took almost a month, but the problem was significantly relieved. The herbs not only worked better than the prescribed drugs, they prevented the need for surgery.

The fourth event occurred when the software company I was working for went bankrupt in 1983. I cast around for new ventures. I was tired of working for others, and wanted to be self-employed. Were I to succeed or fail in the future, it would be by my own hand. Intrigued by acupuncture and herbs, I enrolled in acupuncture college to be my own boss and to learn the mysteries of Chinese medicine.

What I discovered was incredibly simple, but hit me like a shockwave. I learned that following the "laws of nature" will keep you healthy, and that ignoring natural law will make you ill. It sounded so simple, but this truth has staggering effects in real life. The more I learned, the more I realized that traditional Chinese Medicine is a true alternative medicine based on rational principles that have withstood the test of time. I knew the treatments had worked for me, so I resolved to help others as well. I had found my life work.

Now, after twenty-five years of study and practice, having seen countless cures, remissions, and improvements, I want to share my patients' successful experiences with more people. My dual goals are to demystify Chinese medicine and to offer some easy-to-use tools. Many people study Chinese medicine and understand its benefits intellectually, but until it affects your own pain and suffering, you will not be truly persuaded. You do not have to understand the theory to get practical benefits. You just need to be open to the possibility that there is something to be gained from this ancient medicine.

In recent years, China has become a global economic powerhouse. One of China's biggest untapped exports is its wisdom about treating illness based on thousands of years of documented trial-and-error results. Billions of Chinese patients over the millennia have benefited from acupuncture and herbal therapy. These numbers are too large to ignore.

Acupuncture is starting to enter the mainstream in Western countries. Though practiced underground by Chinese immigrants in the United States since the 1800s, America didn't "discover" acupuncture until the early 1970s, when a *New York Times* reporter accompanying President Nixon to China received successful acupuncture treatment during surgery and wrote a column about it. Now, thirty years later, many distinguished Western medical professionals, hospitals, and insurance companies have accepted acupuncture into their overall health care programs.

In contrast, the use of Chinese herbs is not as prevalent as is treatment by acupuncture in the United States. Walk through the Chinatown of a major city and you will see quaint herb shops lined with jars and drawers concealing exotic plants, animals, and God-knows-what. Nothing could seem more foreign, peculiar, or odd. Yet growing numbers of Americans, many initiated by family members and friends, have found enhanced health in these mysterious bottles whiffing these indescribable aromas. We have discovered that there is also logic and method to this strange medicine. Above all, we have found that it works.

I have an audacious vision for this little book: to help many individuals and to assist in streamlining our health care system. Here are two examples of the enormous savings possible with this holistic approach. Over half of all doctor visits in the United States are for upper respiratory ailments, most of which are cold- and flu-related. Were patients to take proven Chinese herbal formulas at the onset of colds and flus, there would be far fewer doctor visits and our medical professionals could redirect their efforts toward treating more serious illnesses. Likewise, quantitative studies have shown that 80 percent of patients with lower back pain who elect to have surgery would have done equally well or better with acupuncture, and at a fraction of the cost. Why go under the knife when there is a proven alternative with 2,500 years of history behind it? When Chinese and Western medicines complement each other, patients benefit from the best of both worlds. I am on a mission to get the word out.

You do not need to be a scholar to learn about and to reap rewards from Chinese medicine. The concepts are simple. We already know them, because we feel them. Chinese medicine is based on what we feel, see, hear, and smell. Once you understand a few simple ideas, you will be more aware of your self and your body. You will become more in tune with how your self and your body interact with the visible and invisible: with mind, matter, and all the laws of nature. The more you understand, the more you can positively influence your health and your recovery from disease.

A Rich Written Tradition

Chinese and Western medicine, unlike oral folk medicines, share a strong written tradition. In the case of Chinese medicine, over 2,000 years of successful diagnosis, treatment, experimentation, and commentary have been meticulously documented.

Seven principal Chinese medicine texts illustrate its rich history.

The earliest book, over 2,500 years old, is the medical text that later became the foundation for Chinese Medicine: *The Yellow Emperor's Inner Classic*, also known as *Plain Questions,* the *Canon of Acupuncture*, and the *Huangdi Neijing.* This work summarizes and systematizes the previous millennia of medical experience and deals with the anatomy and physiology of the human body.

The earliest classic on herbs, *The Herbal*, was handed down from the Qin and Han dynasties (221 BC–220 AD). It discusses 365 kinds of herbs and describes the pharmacological theory and the actions of specific herbal formulations.

The defining text on acupuncture and moxibustion (heat therapy) is *Classic of Acupuncture and Moxibustion*, by Huang Fumi (215–282 AD). It summarizes information on the body channels, therapeutic properties of 349 acupuncture points, needle manipulation, and contraindication.

Diagnosis is the main subject of *Treatise on Febrile Diseases and Miscellaneous Diseases* (300 AD). This classic differentiates febrile diseases according to the theory of six channels, or meridians, distinguishes miscellaneous diseases according to pathological changes of viscera, and establishes diagnosis based on overall analysis of signs and symptoms. Its 269 prescriptions provide the basis for traditional and current clinical practice.

General Treatise on the Causes and Symptoms of Disease (610 AD) is the earliest classic on etiology and syndrome. It lists 1,700 syndromes in sixty-seven categories and expounds on the pathology, signs, and symptoms of various diseases, surgery, gynecology, and pediatrics.

Finally, two classics cover prescriptions. *Prescriptions Worth a Thousand Gold for Emergencies* (581–682 AD) provides 5,300 prescriptions and includes sections on acupuncture, moxibustion, diet therapy, treatment of deficiency diseases, and prevention and health preservation. *The Medical Secrets of an Official* (752 AD) is a master's compendium of 6,000 prescriptions.

How to Use This Book

The next few pages briefly introduce the techniques and principles of Traditional Chinese Medicine (TCM) so you can get familiar with the methods, vocabulary, and holistic philosophy behind the practices. Read as much or as little as you find interesting. I encourage you to spend some time on Chapter 1, "Methods of Chinese Medicine," and Chapter 2, "A Patient's Guide to Acupuncture and Herbs," which together describe the treatment options and responsibilities of both patient and practitioner in achieving optimal results. You don't need to read Chapter 3, "Understanding Theories of Chinese Medicine," to benefit from the subsequent practical sections, but you may find that it stimulates a new way to think about your healing.

After reading Chapter 2, "A Patient's Guide to Acupuncture and Herbs," you are ready to make use of the reference sections of the book: "Treatment of Ailments A to Z" and "Herbs and Their Categories." Look up your health problem or that of someone you know, and learn how this problem is viewed by a practitioner of Traditional Chinese Medicine, or, find a professional in your area. As you become familiar with herb groups, look them up by category to understand the range of ailments they address. This book provides information on both acupuncture and herbal medicine, including the names of herbs and herbal formulas, descriptions, dosages, preparation tips, and information on where to locate the herbs.

A Patient's Guide to Chinese Medicine will help you understand a little of the wisdom and logic of this time-honored medicine. More importantly, it may assist you, your family members, and friends to heal. Whatever the medical condition may be, this book is designed to help you understand it from the perspective of Chinese medicine, then do something about it.

Please keep in mind that the information provided in this book is for educational purposes and is not meant to substitute for the advice of your own physician or other medical professional. I make no claim as to the efficacy or safety of products mentioned in this book. Additionally, information and statements regarding dietary supplements have not been evaluated by the Food and Drug Administration and are not intended to diagnose, treat, cure, or prevent any disease.

I hope you will reach for this handbook often. After all, it is a problem-solving guide for both temporary and persistent conditions. May it bring years of enhanced vigor and harmony to your life.

Acknowledgements and Confessions

Who Is Dr. Shen?

"You mean you're not Chinese?
This changes everything.
I'm not taking advice from a woman who's not Chinese."

—Estelle Costanza of *Seinfeld*

The word *"shen"* is an important medical term used in the practice of Traditional Chinese Medicine. It can mean spirit, mind, or God. Many disorders that in the West are considered "mental" are actually disorders of the spirit, or *shen*.

When my wife Betty and I opened our clinic in 1987, we chose the name "Shen" to distinguish it from conventional clinics of conventional medicine. When our son Noah joined us to market our herbal products, we chose the name Dr. Shen's as a logical outgrowth of our clinic, and because in China all acupuncturists and herbologists are considered and called "doctor." When I began answering medical questions on our website, www.drshen.com, people understandably began calling me Dr. Shen. Despite the risk to my reputation, I must state that my name is not Shen. I am not Chinese, and I am not degreed as a doctor.

My name is Joel Schreck. I grew up in New York City and went to Queens College (the same school as Jerry Seinfeld). I studied acupuncture and Chinese medicine at the now demised San Francisco College of Acupuncture. I have been studying, practicing, and living Traditional Chinese Medicine since 1983. I have also been educated by and thank the following teachers, authors, and true pioneers of Chinese medicine in America: Randall Barolet, Harriet Beinfeld,

Dan Bensky, Yu Min Chen, Misha Cohen, David Eisenberg, Bob Flaws, Larry Forsberg, Jake Fratkin, Jiang Jian Fu, Moon Fung, Andrew Gamble, Robert Johns, Ted Kaptchuck, Efrem Korngold, Robert Levine, Ji Shen, John H. F. Shen, Reese Smith, Jay Tobin, Andrew Tseng, and Robert Zeiger. Above all, thank you Betty and Noah Schreck, for making everything possible with your support, guidance, and hard work.

—Joel Harvey Schreck

1

Methods of
Chinese Medicine

What follows is a brief description of the various components in the Chinese medicine practitioner's toolbox that treat episodic and recurring ailments. Here I introduce acupuncture, moxibustion, massage, bodywork, meditation, movement, martial arts, cupping, and herbal medicine.

Acupuncture

Where there's flow, there's no pain
Chinese Proverb

Acupuncture is a complete medical system that originated in China thousands of years ago. Today it is used throughout the world to treat many different ailments. Acupuncture involves the insertion of hair-thin sterile needles at specific points on the body. Their purpose is to adjust the flow of Qi (vital energy), and thereby influence other nourishing and/or cleansing flows, such as that of blood, lymph, waste, food, hormones, and lubricating fluids. Performed properly, the technique is nearly painless.

How Does It Work?

According to Traditional Chinese Medicine, acupuncture works by promoting or directing the flows of energy and fluids (Qi and blood). These flows nourish the body the same way a farmer irrigates his fields with canals. A farmer regulates water flow via gates. In our bodies, these gates are the acupuncture points. A practitioner stimulates them to help direct this flow of energy.

Numerous controlled studies have shown that acupuncture works for a variety of ailments. Some scientists believe that acupuncture stimulates the nervous system. They theorize that needling affects peripheral nerves, and in turn, that the central nervous system creates far-reaching changes throughout the body by influencing many diverse physiological mechanisms, such as hormonal output, blood production, brain function, respiration, and metabolism. Other studies reveal that acupuncture produces endorphins, morphine-like substances made naturally in the body. Some experts speculate that endorphins may explain the effectiveness of acupuncture.

Moxibustion

Cold is treated with heat
Chinese Medicine Precept

Heat can be beneficial. When the body is cold, it is therapeutic to reintroduce heat. It adds energy back into the body.

Moxibustion is a heat treatment whereby acupuncture points are stimulated by burning an herb called moxa (compressed artemisia leaf) on or near the point. Burning moxa while it sits on the skin is called direct moxibustion. Burning it near the skin is called indirect moxibustion. Sometimes practitioners burn moxa attached to acupuncture needles. This is called Warming Needle Technique.

A moxa stick is like a cigar whose lit tip is burned about an inch from the affected area. When the spot becomes too hot, the moxa stick is withdrawn, then after a moment, it is returned to the point. This is done again and again for five to twenty minutes at a time. You do not need to know acupuncture points to perform moxibustion on yourself; you just need to apply heat to the part of the body that is exhibiting pain. Do it five to twenty minutes per session, one to three sessions per day. Just be careful to not burn the skin, and to ventilate the smoke. Watch for falling ashes, and always extinguish the stick (or roll) by suffocating it in sand, salt, or rice.

Massage and Bodywork

Touch the body, move the Qi
Chinese Medicine Precept

Massage became a precursor of acupuncture when the ancients learned that Qi responded to touch and to the energy of the practitioner. Through millennia of massage treatments and observation, practitioners discovered the channels along which Qi flows and their accompanying acupuncture points.

Asian massage promotes the movement of Qi, blood, and fluids. Tui Na, Shiatsu, and other massage techniques are used for healing and to prevent illness as well as for relaxation. These massage styles differ slightly as they developed in different nations. Shiatsu from Japan, Tui Na in China, and Nuad Bo Rarn, the traditional massage of Thailand, are the most widely known. All may feel similar, varying more by practitioner than by techniques characteristic of a national style. Unlike Swedish massage, they are not langorous and muscle-melting.

Like yin and yang, Asian massage is hard and soft, fast and slow, pleasurable yet slightly painful. Points and channels are stimulated to promote flow. Limbs are stretched and pulled. Sometimes the torso is gently twisted. Patients rarely fall asleep during an invigorating Asian massage treatment.

Meditation, Movement, and Martial Arts

Qi Gong

> *The superior doctor treats when there is no disease*
> Chinese Proverb

Qi Gong (pronounced *chi kung*) is a method of energy cultivation akin to meditation, yet is different. Its objective is to strengthen internal power. It is used to maintain health, increase vitality, prolong life, and expand the mind. In meditation, the mind is cleared and stilled to reach a state of awareness or union with the Absolute, whereas in Qi Gong, the mind is focused on directing energy. Practitioners have a saying for this: "Where the mind goes, energy follows"

Qi Gong is also not the same as creative visualization. In the case of creative visualization, image matter arises in the imagination, existing yet not existing. In the practice of Qi Gong, Qi exists outside the imagination. Qi is considered to be real, palpable, detectable, and subject to manipulation. Qi Gong, therefore, is a much more physical and arguably a more powerful discipline than positive visualization.

Movement and Health

> *The door hinge never rusts*
> Chinese Proverb

Stagnation is the enemy of health. Activity is the great remedy. According to the theory of Traditional Chinese Medicine, movement quickens the blood and scours the vessels, permitting the free flow of blood and Qi. Exercise extends the blood to the smallest vessels, deeply nourishing the body. This same circulation clears waste from every cell. Without proper exercise, the body becomes toxic inside, contaminated by uncleared discharges, and cells wallow in their own waste material. Moderate, regular, vigorous exercise is a foundation for good health, not because it slims the body and tones the muscles, but because it cleans out harmful toxins. It is simply good hygiene.

Tai Chi

> *The journey is the reward*
> Chinese Proverb

Tai Chi (*tai ji*) is a martial arts discipline that can be practiced at any age and has become quite popular in the United States. Its movements are gentle and fluid, not forceful. It is practiced both for self-defense and self-improvement.

Tai Chi improves coordination and helps harmonize the mind and body. Studies show that Tai Chi benefits the body in profound ways: improved mental outlook, better circulation, better immune function, and lower incidence of pain. Studies on senior citizens show that Tai Chi improves balance and prevents falls.

If you decide you want to study Tai Chi, check your yellow pages under "Martial Arts."

Herbal Medicine

> *Speak to the earth,*
> *and it shall teach thee*
> The Bible, Job 22:8

Herbal therapy is estimated to represent 80 percent of the practice of Chinese medicine worldwide. Over 10,000 natural substances are catalogued in the Chinese herbal pharmacopeia. These substances, referred to generically as "herbs," consist of thousands of plant species from all over the world, as well as both mineral and animal materials. Practitioners are referred to as herbologists. Chinese herbs are most often taken in formulas (combinations of herbs) rather than individually. By combining herbs, synergies result that markedly increase the medicinal effects. Blending herbs also allows the herbologist to neutralize unwanted side effects. Traditional formulas consist of principal herbs, assisting herbs, directional herbs, and herbs that reduce side effects or aid the digestion of a particular herb.

Herbs can be ingested as boiled teas called decoctions, milled powders or granules, pills or tablets, extracts, or as steeped tea. Topically, herbs are used in poultices, plasters, soaks, ointments, washes, and fumigants (burning herbs). The "Treatment of Ailments A to Z" reference section of this book describes how you can use herbs at home to improve your overall health.

Decoctions

The potent odors and flavors of Chinese herbs are legendary. Boiling the herbs will provide the fullest medicinal experience of these medicines. Herbs are commonly boiled in ceramic pots for twenty to forty minutes, the dregs are strained out, and the "tea" is taken warm or at room temperature. Boiling times are averaged according to the composition of the formula. Flower and leaf will yield medicine in ten to twenty minutes. Roots take twenty to forty minutes. Shells and minerals must cook for at least one hour. A few herbs, like mint or tangerine peel, must be boiled no more than three to five minutes, lest they loose their valuable volatile oils. These herbs are added separately to the boiling mixture just before completion.

Milled Powders and Granules

Whole herbs can be ground to produce milled powders, or one can purchase pre-packaged powders. They can be boiled, taken as tablets, or steeped in a teabag.

Pills, Tablets, and Capsules

The Chinese invented the pill form of administering medication, which has been used in China since well before the twelfth century. Ancient formulas were often prepared as pills, made from milled herbs bound with water, honey, ginger juice, or other substances. Therapeutic dosages of powders or pills range between three to ten grams daily. The body perceives and responds to herbal medicine much as it does to food, not as it does to a hyper-concentrated chemical pharmaceutical. Think of herbs as ultra-powerful vegetables.

Extracts

The constituents of herbs can be extracted by water, alcohol, vinegar, glycerin, or, in recent times, chemical solvents, to form either granules or tinctures. Most herbologists prefer to use low-temperature whole herb water extraction rather than the extractions used by many modern makers of supplements. Simply soaking an herb in alcohol, vinegar, or glycerin yields tinctures, which are easy to prepare and administer.

Steeped Tea

One of the easiest ways to take herbs is to drop pre-packaged herbal teabags into steaming hot water and let steep for five minutes. This avoids both the ten-to-sixty-minute boiling time and the potent odors of raw herb decoctions.

2

A Patient's Guide to Acupuncture and Herbs

Nature cures the patient,
the doctor collects the fee
Chinese Proverb

Visiting an acupuncturist or a practitioner of Traditional Chinese Medicine is unlike your usual trip to a Western doctor. For those new to this experience, this chapter explains these differences and provides recommendations to get the most out of your trips to acupuncturists and herbologists.

Some dissimilarities are obvious. Practitioners of Traditional Chinese Medicine use unfamiliar techniques, uncommon substances, and reference an unusual philosophy, at least to most Westerners. Do not expect them to have the same training or patient-doctor approach as Western physicians. During your first office visit, ask your practitioner what he or she prefers to be called. Many practitioners prefer to be called doctor, which is the accepted practice in China.

What Patients Expect from Practitioners

According to the philosophy of Traditional Chinese Medicine, above all else, the practitioner will do no harm. The ideal practitioner leads an exemplary life, is indifferent to the wealth of the patient, has compassion for life, and looks upon the patient as if he himself had been stricken. Practitioners of Traditional Chinese Medicine are taught to practice this way and to do their best to achieve these ideals.

The TCM practitioner must be curious about the patient, and will want to know about his/her life. Disease is rooted in the patient's experiences, so the practitioner must be a detective, sifting through signs, symptoms, and clues to solve the disease and restore harmony to the patient. The practitioner may administer herbs or acupuncture, or consult philosophical principles to illuminate the cause and permit the cure. The Four Examinations are used to diagnose the patient.

The Four Examinations

1. Looking
The practitioner observes the patient's body tone, gait, skin, facial expression, emotional tone, and mannerisms. He or she also examines the tongue, with the heart condition shown at the tip and the kidneys at the root, according to TCM theory. The tongue's color and coating show what may be hidden, revealing hot from cold, damp from dry, and excess from deficient.

2. Listening
The TCM practitioner must be attentive to the patient's story and history, and must put aside preconceptions. The practitioner listens to the patient's voice, noting its volume and clarity, manner of speaking, and use of language. The voice can also reveal ailments.

3. Smelling and Tasting
The TCM practitioner may ask about body odors and tastes. Smells and tastes are clues. Strong tastes and odors can be signs of heat, toxicity, or digestive stagnation.

4. Touching

The practitioner feels the pulse on both wrists. Besides noting its rate, rhythm, and overall strength, a TCM practitioner will note the quality of the pulse. It is difficult to express in words what is meant by "quality of the pulse." Detecting the pulse is an art that is challenging to master, yet once mastered rewards the practitioner with the ability to sense something of the internal condition of the patient. The patient may not tell the truth, but the pulse never lies. To guide practitioners to feel the pulse, the ancients defined twenty-eight types. Some common types are:

Wiry feels tense, like a bowstring

Thready feels thin and narrow

Deep strong pressure required to feel it

Short slow and irregular

Slippery feels like a bubble moving

The practitioner may also touch the body. Local sensitivity can reveal what needs attention. The practitioner might feel for skin or muscle tone, temperature, sensitivity, unhealthy accumulations, or other signs of abnormality.

Whereas an M.D. is more interested in your lab tests than your perceptions, a practitioner of Traditional Chinese Medicine has the opposite point of view. Physicians of the Ming dynasty did not have lab tests; they learned to pay careful attention to their patients' signs and symptoms. They learned from study, personal experience, and the wisdom of their elders and ancestors. Through careful observation and trial and error, they discovered ways for people to cure themselves through natural means.

Chinese medicine diagnosis is based entirely on what you, the patient, show, tell, and exude (e.g., voice qualities) about yourself. Your collection of complaints, your countenance, posture, voice, pulse, and life story—together form a unique pattern. By comparing your pattern with others observed, noted, and described over millennia, the TCM practitioner forms a preliminary diagnosis. Equipped with this assessment, numerous therapeutic alternatives (acupuncture, moxibustion, massage), and a plethora of herbal medicines, the practitioner charts a course of treatment.

Accreditation and Kinds of Practitioners

Be sure to check the background practitioners, because there are many acupuncturists who do not practice the complete science. In the United States and Europe, most Chinese medicine professionals are acupuncturists, but not all acupuncturists are practitioners of Traditional Chinese Medicine. Learning the skills of diagnosis and herbal prescription takes much longer than learning the basic placement of acupuncture needles.

Unfortunately, point location is the only skill a candidate for licensure must demonstrate in order to practice acupuncture in most states. Except in New Mexico, Western medical doctors have unlimited rights to use needles and need not demonstrate any acupuncture knowledge or skills to practice acupuncture. As a group, such MDs are called Medical Acupuncturists. Although there are many notable exceptions, many MD acupuncturists receive their training in China through fast-track courses such as the one offered by the China Beijing Acupuncture Training Center, which offers certification for a total of 400 hours of training. This includes theory, location of 120 points (out of about 500), and clinical practice. These courses are designed to teach the basics and do not necessarily turn out skilled or experienced acupuncturists.

Most acupuncture practitioners in the United States have little training in Chinese medicine. They are usually trained as chiropractors, MDs, or naturopathic or homeopathic physicians. Most have little or no skill in Chinese diagnostic techniques, or in the intricacies of prescribing Chinese herbs. An acupuncturist's affinity for Chinese medicine or lack thereof is probably apparent, as those who are currently seeing one know. When choosing a practitioner, inquire about his or her formal training and orientation.

When you investigate your potential practitioner's qualifications, you will discover an assortment of initials and credentials. Each country has its own standards concerning the practice of acupuncture and herbal medicine. Within the United States, each state sets its own qualifications for licensed acupuncturists. Acupuncturists have "primary care physician" status in California and New Mexico, and are required to pass state board examinations covering Western medicine, Chinese herbal medicine, and acupuncture. Most other states recognize passing the National Committee for the Certification of Acupuncture and Oriental Medicine (NCCAOM) examination as a standard for acupuncture licensure.

The qualifications to practice herbal medicine are unregulated in America. Less widespread in use than acupuncture in the United States, the field of herbal medicine lacks the special attention and financing needed for lawmakers to create and pass state legislation. The NCCAOM offers a separate examination for Chinese herbal medicine that excludes acupuncture. However, no state requires practitioners to pass the herbal exam to practice. Since herbal therapy is the most commonly practiced method of Chinese medicine in the world, the public health is better served and protected when states adopt the NCCAOM herbal exam as a licensing standard for those intending to practice Chinese herbal medicine.

Most practitioners of alternative medicine who have discovered the power of Chinese herbs gain competence by practicing on their patients. I am no exception. Consumers should be cognizant of the varied degree of herbal or medical experience of their practitioner. In addition to herbalists, who are usually the most qualified to prescribe herbs, acupuncturists, MDs, chiropractors, naturopaths, massage therapists, and even the clerk at the health food store do so as well.

Because acupuncture is considered a medical procedure, educational requirements for acupuncturists are more established. However, the variety of initials after acupuncturists' names needs to be decoded. Accreditations behind the most prevalent titles are:

CA Certified Acupuncturist. An acupuncture school has granted this person a certificate of completion. School programs vary in their offerings from 200 to 2,000 hours of training. Some school programs include herbal medicine training, and others do not. The Certified Acupuncturist certificate is not a license to practice.

LAc Licensed Acupuncturist. This is a license to practice (and is the title I hold). These practitioners have passed state board examinations. In California and New Mexico, such acupuncturists are regulated as primary care physicians (PCP); you can use them as your doctor. They can order lab tests, do physical exams, accept insurance (when it covers acupuncture), and handle Worker's Compensation cases. Acupuncturists cannot perform surgery. They can prescribe only "drugless substances," which refers to natural herbs, not manufactured pharmaceutical chemicals.

OMD, DOM Doctor of Oriental Medicine. Oriental medicine is similar to Chinese medicine but includes practices from other Asian countries as well. You see these letters frequently, but their meaning is not straightforward. They do not connote a license to practice. Rather, they indicate a doctoral degree offered by an accredited school. Only a handful of accredited OMD or DOM degree programs operate in the United States. However, the state of New Mexico allows its certified acupuncturists to use OMD by their names without the required advanced degree training, thus diluting the legitimacy of this title.

MD China Medical Doctor in China. This degree permits medical practice only in China. These physicians, trained in Western medicine in China, are not allowed to practice Western medicine in the United States without further accreditation. Hence, many open Chinese medicine clinics. However, the title MD China does not indicate any formal training in Chinese medicine, though certain individuals may be so trained.

Dipl. Ac. Diplomate in Acupuncture, and **Dipl. Herb** Diplomate in Herbology. The bearers of these initials have passed the NCCAOM (National Committee for the Certification of Acupuncture and Oriental Medicine) examination, and are members of the NCCAOM. There are separate exams for acupuncture and herbs. Though not a license, this acupuncture test is used by many states as a qualifying exam. The

NCCAOM lists the following requirements for certification:

1. Must be at least eighteen years of age.
2. Must complete the eligibility requirements through formal education or apprenticeship. Formal Education: must graduate from a full-time acupuncture program with at least 1,725 hours of acupuncture education, with a minimum of 1,000 didactic and 500 clinical hours. Apprenticeship: must complete an apprenticeship of at least 4,000 patient contact hours within a three to six year period.
3. Must successfully complete a Clean Needle Technique (CNT) course approved by the NCCAOM.
4. Must sign a statement agreeing to be bound by the National Code of Ethics of the NCCAOM.
5. Must pass the NCCAOM Acupuncture Examination consisting of the Comprehensive Written Examination in Acupuncture, and the Point Location Examination.

Fulfilling these requirements permits eligibility in about forty states. California and New Mexico have separate, more demanding requirements, especially in Western medicine and herbal medicine, because acupuncturists in those states have the status of primary care physicians.

What Practitioners Expect from Patients

Chinese medicine requires more dedication from the patient than does Western medicine. Many people are accustomed to spending a few minutes with the doctor and taking a prescribed pill for ailments. For some patients, Chinese medicine requires nothing more than a visit to the acupuncturist and lying passively on the treatment table. However, for many patients, Chinese medicine requires a greater investment in time to cover acupuncture treatments, herb preparation and administration, meditation, exercise, and doing other activities to harmonize your life. For those with chronic or serious afflictions, Chinese medicine can become a life-changing experience.

Moreover, practitioners expect the patient to be the teacher. Nobody knows you like you do. According to Chinese medicine theory, nobody can heal you but yourself. While the practitioner has had many teachers, the patient is always the greatest teacher. Patients will learn to know and understand what the practitioner needs to know about them—and to distinguish that from what is less relevant.

Diagnosis and treatment are based on a practitioner's perceptions of you and your complaints. A TCM practitioner observes you, listens to you, examines your tongue, and feels your pulse. A good practitioner sees the obvious, yet depends on you to explain how you feel, or to reveal other symptoms that are below the surface. A practitioner is interested in your perceptions and visualizations concerning your condition, and your view of its cause.

Practitioners need to know about all your complaints, not just the ones you came in with. For example, if you made an appointment for lower back pain, it is important for the practitioner to know if you are also tired, have achy knees, or whether your extremities are hot or cold. If a headache brought you to the practitioner's clinic, the rash on your buttocks might be the best clue to relieving your headache.

A TCM practitioner also must know all the medicines and supplements you are taking, not just the ones for your chief complaint. Herbs rarely interfere with drugs; there are, however, a few combinations that should be avoided. Taking blood-vitalizing herbs together with blood-thinning drugs could cause bleeding and is taboo. Taking strong heat-clearing herbs with antibiotics could overstress digestion and cause diarrhea. Taking herbs with poisonous or extremely cold properties together with toxic chemotherapy agents should also be avoided. Knowing about your full course of prescribed and over-the-counter medicine, as well as other supplements you are taking, will influence what may or may not be recommended for you.

Teach your practitioner about your preferences and concerns. Do you have strong positive or negative positions regarding your treatment? "I love acupuncture," "I fear needles," "I gag on pills," "I'm concerned about the safety of herbs." Practitioners need to know this information to chart a smooth course of treatment that provides enough time, energy, and inclination for you to follow it.

Provide the TCM practitioner with your complete medical history. I recall an acupuncture patient who came in for chronic insomnia and mentioned no other complaints during the interview, in spite of repeated requests. When performing the acupuncture treatment, I asked him about the enormous scar I saw on his chest. "Quadruple bypass last year," he answered. He did not know that, in Chinese medicine, insomnia is intricately related to the heart.

Your medical doctor's diagnosis of your condition may not be relevant to practitioners of Chinese medicine. Almost everyone who comes to me for the first time has previously seen an MD or chiropractor. I can learn something about you and your condition by knowing what you have already tried, and what has worked or not worked in the past. TCM practitioners rely on their own comprehensive system of diagnosis to set expectations and direct a course of treatment.

The Western medical diagnosis of arthritis is a case in point. Arthritis means joint pain, and diagnosing it does not require the skills of a highly trained professional. A typical arthritis diagnosis is discouraging, as arthritis is considered a degenerative disease with no cure. The patient sees no hope of improvement, despairs, and expects the condition to worsen. To practitioners of Traditional Chinese Medicine, however, an arthritis diagnosis simply means that the flow in the joint is impaired. This could be due to an old injury, a weakening of defensive energy, a systemic problem with flow, or other causes. To Chinese medical practitioners, these problems are treatable.

Stay the Course

How long will it take? The practitioner cannot be sure at first. In general, the older the condition is, the longer its course of treatment. For some acute problems, results can occur immediately. Recently sprained ankles often feel better and heal noticeably after a single acupuncture treatment. Yin Chiao tablets and other Chinese cold medicines work within an hour. Stomach Curing Pills relieve nausea within ten minutes. Superior Sore

Throat Powder eases pain instantly, upon application.

Chronic, long-term, or recurring ailments are naturally more complicated, more difficult to treat, and require patience. Chinese medicine is neither a miracle nor a panacea. When the condition is difficult for Western medicine, it may also be difficult for Traditional Chinese Medicine. Sometimes improvement is all that can be expected. Sometimes only stabilization is possible. It may be helpful for chronically ill people to see wellness as a destination that is distant, yet in plain sight. There are bumps and twists and turns along the way, but, like a traveler on a winding road, one is making progress.

A rule of thumb is that it takes a month of treatment for every year the disorder was present or incubating. A five-year ailment may take as long as five months to resolve, if indeed resolution is possible, but patients may get partial relief much sooner. Though it is difficult to predict with certainty, Chinese medicine usually assists most people within six visits. If they show no signs of improvement after six visits, I probably will not be able to help them with acupuncture. Some people will not come six times if they did not notice a benefit early on, and will quit too soon.

It is not uncommon for people to come for only a single treatment. When that one treatment does not produce a noticeable result, they move on to something else. Even when treatment helps, patients sometime stop too soon. The most common reason patients cancel appointments is not because the condition did not improve, but rather because they feel better and do not want to pay for an unnecessary visit. The traditional course of treatment is usually double the amount of time it takes to eliminate symptoms. For example, when your sciatica symptoms disappear after three weeks, your course of treatment should extend another three weeks to prevent recurrence.

Herbal Pointers

There are many ways to take Chinese herbs—pills, powders, plasters, tinctures, decoctions, tonics, and teas. I find that Chinese herbs are extremely reliable for many different conditions. When the herbs are not working after being properly prescribed, the problem is usually not with the herbs, but with the patient. The mistakes most new patients make are either to not take enough medicine or to not communicate with their practitioner. Fear about taking these unfamiliar substances, coupled with the large dosages sometimes required, causes many to take lower amounts than needed. Though some people can get results with smaller amounts, it is far better to take the traditional dose, which has been determined by generations of trial and error.

Nonetheless, when you find it difficult to take a large amount of herbs, or when the herbs are not working as expected, communicate, do not quit. Consult your practitioner. He or she may advise a different method of administration or a different dose. Do not be restricted by a method of administration that doesn't work for you. I have seen too many people stop taking Chinese herbs just because they were forced to boil and drink them. In most cases, the key to success is perseverence, so it is important to find the most comfortable way to take your herbs.

How to Take Pills

"Why so many?" new patients exclaim in disbelief, after I tell them to take twenty-four pills a day. Herbs are different than manufactured pharmaceuticals. Most herbal pills consist of ground-up roots, bark, leaves, and other plant material. A good part of this is fiber, which adds significantly to the volume of the herbal medicine. Even herbal concentrates, which have been extracted from the plant's fiber, must still be taken in much larger amounts than many are accustomed to.

Pharmaceutical chemicals are toxic in large amounts. Herbs contain only tiny amounts of these chemicals, and herbal forumulas also contain many additional ingredients to buffer the effects of the herbs. While all this often makes herbs safer than equivalent pharmaceuticals, it may require larger doses.

So, when you want Chinese herbs to work as well or better than pharmaceutical products, you may need to get used to consuming four to forty pills a day. Pill sizes can vary from 200 to 800 miligrams. Thirty 200-gram pills yield only six grams of medicine per day. That is about two tablespoons, less than the amount of sugar found in a bottle of soda.

What to Take with Pills

Most patients take pills on an empty stomach two to three times a day, a regimen recommended for most conditions. Taking pills on an empty stomach increases absorption of the medicine up to 30 percent. Practitioners most often recommend taking pills with warm or room-temperature water. However, other liquids can be used for special circumstances. For kidney ailments, herbal pills can be taken with salt water to increase action upon the kidney. Herbs for injury are frequently taken with alcohol to better move the blood and break stagnations. Herbs for stomach problems can be made more digestible when taken with sweet liquids.

How to Drink Decoctions

Some patients enjoy drinking herbal blends as tea, but, for many people, effective doses of some medicinal herbs have an unpleasant taste, and cooking these herbs can smell up your kitchen or house. Remember to always boil herbs in a pot made of ceramic, heat-resistant glass, or stainless steel. Never use aluminum or iron cookware to boil or heat herbs; when heated, these two metals will readily leach from the cookware, recombine with chemicals in the medicine, and alter the chemical composition of the brew.

Follow this preparation and consumption tip list: 1) While cooking herbs, ventilate the kitchen. 2) Hold your nose when you drink unpleasant-tasting herbs. This eliminates almost all of the taste. 3) Drink herbs with lukewarm water to help your body absorb the medicine. Sipping hot liquids slowly, as one has to, unnecessarily extends the unpleasantness. Cold liquids have less taste but do not digest as well as lukewarm preparations. 4) Chew a few raisins or place a drop of lemon juice on your tongue after swallowing to eliminate any aftertaste.

Like pills, herbal decoctions usually work best when taken on an empty stomach. Allow at least a half hour after taking herbs before eating or swallowing additional medicines. When the medicine proves difficult to digest even with warm water, take it with food or after a meal. Some practitioners believe that formulas designed for the upper body should be taken after eating. Other medicines are best taken with liquids such as wine (injuries or vascular problems), date broth (to aid digestion of the herbs), or salt water (messenger to the kidneys).

How to Take Tinctures and Elixirs

Tinctures are generally alcohol extracts. However, vinegar, glycerin, and other solvents are sometimes used to dissolve the chemical components and separate these active constituents from fibrous herbal material. Tinctures are best diluted with a small amount of water to reduce the effect of the alcohol they contain. Heating these liquids can evaporate some of the alcohol. Herbal wines, on the other hand, intentionally contain alcohol to move the blood, and are especially useful for injury and in old age. Western medicine has recently discovered what the Chinese have known for a thousand years—that a little wine is bad for pregnant women and good for the health of older people.

How to Take Milled Powders and Granules

Whole herbs are ground up and sifted to produce milled powders. Once they have been milled, herbs can then be formed into tablets, poured into capsules, or put into a teabag to be boiled and steeped.

Granules, on the other hand, are extracts made from herbs that have been pre-boiled. These extracts are often referred to as freeze-dried herbs, although they are actually spray dried. Boiled-down herbal liquids are sprayed on a water-soluble medium such as corn starch, rice starch, or simple sugar. The resulting powder can be dissolved in water before administration. Granules of individual herbs can easily be combined into formulas that will dissolve in water. Dissolving granulated formulas in water is much quicker and easier than boiling herbal decoctions. They often have a pungent taste. Granules have become popular in Taiwan, Japan, and the United States, but not in China, where people still prefer to boil their herbs.

Use as much water as you like to dissolve the granules. I prefer to drink no more than a quarter of a cup of medicine, so I use a small amount of steaming hot water to dissolve the granules. Generally, the hotter the water, the better they dissolve. Let them cool or add a little cold water. I stir in an ice cube to get instant room-temperature herbs without a lot of extra liquid to drink.

California Proposition 65 Warning Labels

For readers who buy Chinese herbs in California and for those who purchase them from California-based providers, here is some information about California's Proposition 65.

When purchasing Chinese herbal medicines in a California natural food store, you may notice a curious warning on the label that states the product "contains substances known by the state of California to cause cancer, birth defects, or other reproductive harm." It sounds harsh, but rest assured, these products are safe. Trace amounts of lead are the issue. Although there is a general consensus that excessive lead can be harmful, regulatory agencies disagree on the appropriate levels for herbal products. Japan allows twenty parts per million for total metals in herbal medicines. The World Health Organization allows ten parts per million of lead in a product, and Germany and the Australian TGA allow five. The U.S. Pharmacopeia has no standards for herbs, but allows three parts per million in drugs. Most Chinese herbal products test at an average of one to three. However, California's Proposition 65 requires warnings at only 0.5 parts per million. This level is ten times lower than any previously established.

California Proposition 65, also known as the California Safe Drinking Water and Toxic Enforcement Act, was enacted in 1986. One of its many provisions restricted the amount of heavy metals allowed in food and water. Though these elements are pervasive in nature and occur naturally in food and water, excessive exposure can cause birth defects and some kinds of cancers. This controversial California law was intended for food and water, not herbal medicine. Herbal medicines are legally considered to be food, and therefore are under the rule of Proposition 65. If they were classified as a medicine, herbal products would fall under the regulatory control of the federal government, whose standards would allow six times the lead made standard under Proposition 65.

Standards used for food and water set an unrealistic level to achieve for authentic herbal medicines that come from the earth and are rich in naturally occurring minerals. Proposition 65 allows the sale of herbal products as long as they carry cautionary labels. California residents are not usually disturbed by these labels, as they appear in every grocery and liquor store, warning us of the dangers present in our food. Rest assured that most of these products meet internationally accepted standards for herbal medicines. Please do not be dissuaded from using them.

Acupuncture Pointers

If you have never had acupuncture, you may have questions before taking the plunge. You might wonder what the needles feel like and if they hurt when inserted. You may have heard conflicting reports from friends and acquaintances. Some say it does not hurt, others say just a little. Acupuncture is almost painless when administered correctly. It would not have survived generations of public acceptance if the needles caused pain. Acupuncture points are free of nerves and blood vessels, so treatment should not cause pain or bleeding. However, it is common and appropriate for your body to respond to the needles with a mild ache, a sense of numbness, or a slight tingle.

A basic experience of acupuncture treatment is the sensation that the needles produce when inserted at certain acupuncture points. This is called obtaining Qi. Though not painful, this sensation is sometimes described as "sore," "numb," "achy," or "heavy." Often the acupuncturist will manipulate the needles until you feel this sensation. When this sensation is perceived, Qi has been obtained, and a positive therapeutic outcome is possible.

Usually, the acupuncturist will not rely on the patient's perception to know when Qi has been obtained. The practitioner can usually feel your muscle tissue "grip" the needle as it is gently manipulated. This indicates that the Qi has "arrived." In some cases of weakness or damage, a needling sensation cannot be obtained immediately. In those instances, the needle can be reintroduced at a different location or at a different angle, or another attempt to obtain Qi is made later, after the Qi has had time to consolidate at the chosen point.

When a patient experiences extreme or sustained pain, that means the needle is off its mark, and must be withdrawn or adjusted. Though several points are known to cause a more intense sensation when needled, treatment should be comfortable. When it isn't, ask your practitioner to deal with it immediately. Besides the feel of the needles, patients report other sensations. For most, the experience is quite relaxing. Many fall asleep. Some fall into a pleasant trance, or experience various flows of energy throughout their body. I have found that what a patient experiences during an acupuncture session may have nothing to do with the medical outcome. The earth may move and the skies open, but symptoms may persist. About half of my patients feel some relief immediately after treatment. Others feel nothing during initial treatment, but feel better the next day or after several treatments. In some cases, I was unable to assist at all.

On occasion, a patient experiences unexpected relief or improvement for a condition unrelated to the one undergoing treatment. I cannot count the number of times people have come for treatment of pain, but then report improvements in their energy, sleep, outlook, or disposition.

Practical Suggestions

Wear loose-fitting clothing for acupuncture. Practitioners often needle the extremities. Some of the most powerful acupuncture points are near the ankles, knees, wrists, and elbows. It is much easier to roll up your cuffs or sleeves than to take off your clothing. When you feel more comfortable without outer clothes, request a dressing gown, and ask whether the front or back should be open.

Go to the bathroom first. Practitioners want you to feel fully relaxed; acupuncture will help you calm down, but not when nature's calling.

For the two hours before or after an acupuncture treatment, I discourage sex, drugs, alcohol, or strenuous exercise. These activities can dissipate and disorder the Qi, minimizing the effect of treatment.

After inserting the needles, most acupuncturists will make sure that you are comfortable, then leave the room and allow you to be alone. If you feel nervous or insecure about being left alone, especially during the first treatment, ask for a bell or other method of getting the acupunturist's attention.

Do not be afraid to tell your MD about your Chinese medicine treatment. You do not require a doctor's permission to see an acupuncturist in most states. Herbologist visits are not regulated in any state. Most MDs are non-committal about acupuncture and suspicious about herbs, which is understandable based on their Western training. It is impossible to fathom and appreciate Chinese medicine through a purely Western lens. I would not consider the average American medical doctor sufficiently educated about Chinese medicine to form a credible opinion. One patient told me that her doctor forbade her to take the herbs I had prescribed during her cancer treatment despite the relief they provided for the side effects of radiation.

Your Western doctor may not be interested in Chinese medicine, but do tell him/her when you are under care. Treatment with Chinese medicine should not concern other practitioners you may be seeing, but it is good for them to know about your experiences with acupuncture and herbs.

Cost of Treatment

The cost of acupuncture and herbs depends largely on supply and demand. I practice in the San Francisco Bay Area, which has a high cost of living. Yet acupuncture in San Francisco is far less expensive than it is in most parts of the United States because so many acupuncturists practice in this region. In most places of the country, I estimate that the ratio between acupuncturists and the general population is one acupuncturist to 50,000 citizens. In the Bay Area, by contrast, which is home to three acupuncture colleges and where acupuncture has become popular, the ratio is about one acupuncturist to 2,000. This plethora of practitioners in the Bay Area has been good for consumers; the cost of acupuncture here can be as little as half of what it costs elsewhere. Treatment costs vary from as low as one fifth (school teaching clinics) to the same as a typical office visit to an MD for a private session. Before deciding on a practitioner, call several in your area to inquire about pricing.

The price may also depend on your willingness to negotiate. Many practitioners of Chinese medicine will negotiate their fees because their lower office overhead and smaller insurance costs allow more flexibility. Others are motivated to expand the practice of Chinese medicine to wider audiences, or will respond to your special circumstances. Others will not negotiate. But you will never know if you could have received treatment for a reduced rate unless you ask.

Compared to the cost of Western technological medicine, Chinese medicine is a bargain. However, when patients already pay expensive health insurance premiums, alternative medicines are sometimes an added financial burden. Most insurance policies do not cover acupuncture, although an increasing number do. Coverage varies considerably by company and state, and is subject to change each year. In California, nonprofit insurance companies (the majority) are required by law to offer at least one policy covering acupuncture. No matter what state you live in, ask your health insurance company which policies cover acupuncture. The more frequently these companies hear requests for acupuncture, the more probable they will offer coverage soon. You can also ask about Chinese herbs, but because herbal medicine lacks the licensing and legal status of acupuncture (specialized needles are FDA-approved medical devices), it is unlikely to be a covered benefit in the foreseeable future.

Find out early in the process whether you or your insurance company will pay the bills. When insurance companies pay, patients seldom consider the cost. Most acupuncturists request payment at the time of treatment. My clinic accepts credit cards, but not all practitioners provide this service. You may want to ask before your first visit. When you have insurance that does cover acupuncture, give the practitioner your insurance information on the phone before the first visit. This enables the claim to be verified first. Though verification does not insure that the claim will be paid, it helps. While verifying eligibility, the practitioner can determine the details of the insurance company's policies concerning acupuncture. These details may differ widely and provide the insurance company with a rationale for non-payment. For example, one firm might only pay for chronic or acute problems, while another may only cover acupuncture treatment as a surgical anesthetic. Many insurance companies routinely reject claims, arguing that acupuncture is not covered for your particular ailment. To avoid most of these rejections, make sure that whatever your reasons are for seeking acupuncture, you are also treated for pain.

Be sure to get a record of your treatment. Acupuncture is a medical treatment and a legitimate income tax deduction. Also, ask if your practitioner will file an insurance claim for you. Though most MDs do this routinely, few acupuncturists have the office staff to deal with insurance billing or the administrative bureaucracy of insurance companies. Acupuncturists will usually give you a "super bill" containing all the information your insurance company will need to process the claim. You must then file the claim yourself.

Chinese Medicine in the United States

The U.S. health care system is threatened by the spiraling cost of services, technology, and drugs. I see patients regularly who avoid visiting their doctor because they cannot afford it. Some are uninsured; others have high deductible policies that do not cover routine or diagnostic visits.

I believe that Chinese medical therapies can actually become the salvation of our health care system, providing safe, inexpensive treatment as well as preventive therapies, thus reducing the cost of many routine and chronic illnesses so prevalent in society.

Common colds account for over 50 percent of doctor visits. Unfortunately, your doctor can do very little to treat colds. Indeed, antibiotics over-prescribed for colds do harm as the body builds resistance to them, making it harder to fight more serious infections that require these powerful drugs.

Most people who have used traditional Chinese cold remedies agree that Chinese medicine is particularly effective for this common ailment. These herbs relieve symptoms quickly and reliably, and they do so without making one groggy, edgy, or affecting consciousness in any way. Scores of these Chinese cold remedies, many with proven anti-viral properties, work better than over-the-counter pharmaceutical drugs.

Unfortunately, this is still a well-kept secret in the West, and doctors' waiting rooms are still routinely filled with sniffling, sneezing patients. If all these head cold sufferers suddenly became enlightened and took *yin chiao* or *gan mao ling* instead of spending half a day waiting around for a doctor's prescription, our physicians would have much more time to focus on more serious medical illnesses or spend more than five minutes with each patient.

If doctors had only half as many patients, perhaps the adjusted supply and demand would lower the cost of an office visit for everyone. Competition is supposed to keep prices low, but Western medicine presently lacks true competition. As Chinese medicine becomes more popular, my hope is that it may act as a competitive catalyst that will actually force prices down, making doctor visits, and ultimately all medical procedures, more affordable for all.

3

Understanding Theories of Chinese Medicine

The theory of Chinese medicine states that human body processes are interrelated and are in continual interaction with nature and the environment. Symptoms, complaints, and physical signs help practitioners diagnose, treat, and assist the patient to heal. The principles are used as a framework by acupuncture and herbal therapy practitioners to understand the patient, the disease pattern, and the way through. When interviewing a patient, the Traditional Chinese Medicine practitioner draws upon the perspective of several fundamental theories to better understand your condition.

Qi and Blood

Flow and Movement

> *Qi is the origin of movement and the source of heat*
> Chinese Medicine precept

Qi (pronounced *chee*) is life force or life energy. It is the sum of all your body's electrical, chemical, magnetic, and radiant energies. Indeed, Qi is the foundation upon which everything else in Chinese medicine builds. TCM practitioners study where it comes from, where it goes, and how it flows. Your body is nourished by, cleansed by, and dependent upon the flow of Qi.

Qi must flow for bodies to stay healthy. Movement shows that Qi exists and warmth shows that Qi is present. Qi and blood nourish the body. Chinese medicine theory states that Qi moves the blood, and blood is mother of the Qi. Normal flows of Qi and blood are the basics of good health. When they are abundant and flowing, the body is well. When blood or Qi is weak, stuck, or flowing improperly, the body becomes ill.

Yin and Yang

Balance, Harmony, and Change

> *You can't argue with nature,*
> *it is always 100 percent correct*
> Chinese Proverb

If Qi is the primary energy, yin and yang are the balance, harmony, and change in life. Yin and yang originally denoted opposite sides of a mountain. In the morning, one side was in shade, the other in sunlight. Later in the day, the sides reversed. Dark became light and light turned to dark. Yin and yang describe the continuous force of change and the intertwined nature of things. Yin and yang also symbolize balance and harmony in our perpetual interplay with the rest of nature.

Yin and yang relationships are more than just opposites. They support and require each other. Indeed, yin and yang also include one another. There is always yin within yang and yang within yin. The traditional, circular yin-yang symbol shows the interrelated nature of yin and yang, where each flows into the next and each has a component of the other within.

Examples of yin and yang are all around. Seemingly opposite forces bind with each other: male and female, hot and cold, down and up, inside and outside, day and night, front and back, upper and lower.

Think of the undercurrent that pulls a bodysurfer away from shore. Now think of riding a wave back to shore. The vibrating water of the oceans is a natural ebb and flow. Nature is full of varying wave lengths, of vibration. Visualize Qi as the moving wave, with regular amplitude and frequency. Now imagine yin and yang as different dimensions of how the wave moves and oscillates.

Yin and Yang Examples

Yang	Yin
Hot	Cold
Activity	Rest
Upper body	Lower body
Outer body	Inner body
Acute diseases	Chronic diseases
Excess conditions	Deficient conditions

Practitioners of Traditional Chinese Medicine see the body and its disharmonies in changing shades of yin and yang. When yin or yang dominates, disharmony results. This affects the course of Qi, and leads to physical and/or mental disharmony. Paying attention to yin and yang helps assess balance and harmony, and also aids practitioners in understanding a disease and a patient.

The Eight Principles

Locate Disease and Understand its Nature

> Location, location
> Chinese Proverb

Chinese medicine relies on the Eight Principles to assess the location and nature of an illness. These eight are four yin-yang pairs of conditions—excess/deficient, inside/outside, hot/cold, and damp/dry. Once these are known, the TCM practitioner formulates the appropriate treatment plan, such as strengthening weakness, cooling heat, or moistening dryness, to rebalance the body.

Excess/Deficient

These terms describe too much or too little of some component of nature. It can describe both the disease and the patient. Sudden illness comes from excess. Chronic illness suggests deficiency. Symptoms of excess are stronger or more pronounced than those caused by deficiency. A severe sore throat suggests wind-heat excess (viral and yang), while a persistent scratchy throat implies heat caused by a deficiency of coolness (yin).

Inside/Outside

Practitioners ask where the disharmony originates. Is it invading from outside the body, or is it caused by deficiency, emotion, or stagnation inside the body? Airborne viruses, bacterial infections, or other pestilential diseases are exterior. Exterior diseases can penetrate the body and become interior diseases. Examples include an airborne disease such as strep throat turning into rheumatic fever, or food- and water-borne organisms breeching defenses, penetrating deep into the body to cause serious harm to the organs, as with hepatitis or cholera. Knowing the nature and location of the pathogenic invader helps the practitioner prescribe the right treatment.

Hot/Cold

Hot/cold pairing is not primarily related to temperature. In this pathology, heat means overstimulation or hyperactivity, and may or may not be reflected in body temperature. Heat suggests an oversupply of Qi or an inadequacy in the body's cooling system. Cold suggests the opposite: understimulation, poor flow, Qi deficiency, or weak metabolic function. Just as it can be hot in Florida while cold in Siberia, bodies too can be hot and cold at the same time. The liver can be hot while the kidney is cold. Diseases can also have hot or cold natures, depending on the way they affect the body. TCM practitioners can spot hot/cold imbalances and help the patient to bring them back into harmony.

Damp/Dry

All life loves water, and that includes viruses, bacteria, and especially fungus. Excessive dampness inside the body helps this microscopic life to breed. Swollen tissue, excess phlegm, or other excess fluids are signs of dampness. Dryness demonstrates a scarcity of fluids, often not only in the skin, but also throughout the body. Dryness can be caused by blood or yin deficiency. Excessive heat can also scorch the fluids and lead to dryness. Prolonged exposure to dry weather leads to dryness inside the body as well as outside.

The Fourteen Channels

Where there's pain, there's no flow
Chinese Proverb

Qi energy travels along fourteen major channels and numerous minor channels. The channels (also called meridians) are segments of one continuous flow that begins at the tips of the fingers and travels upward to the head and face. From there, the Qi then flows down the back and sides to the tips of the toes where it next rises from the feet to nourish the groin, belly, and chest. Issuing from the chest, the Qi then flows outward through the arms, completing the cycle at the tips of the fingers.

These flows influence the fluids and energies in the body. Each segment of this river of energy penetrates an internal organ and is named according to it. Each half of the body has channels named for the lungs, large intestine, stomach, spleen, heart, small intestine, urinary bladder, kidney, pericardium, gallbladder, and liver. In addition, two channels run up the center of the body and meet in the head. The Conception Vessel runs up the front of the body from the perineum to the head, where it meets the Governing Vessel, which runs up the spine from the anus to the head. To the acupuncturist, approximately 500 points along the channels/meridians provide access to the internal organs.

Acupuncture involves placing one or more fine needles into the skin at predetermined points to generate a therapeutic response. Many people receiving acupuncture for the first time are surprised by where the needles are placed. Often they are placed in the extremities, with motives that seem less than obvious. Patients who suffer headaches, for example, find themselves with needles in their hands and feet.

Acupuncture points, like faucets, are used to regulate flow along these channels. The most powerful points on these channels lie on the extremities, below the elbows and below the knees. Five powerful points on the extremity of each channel are known as the five "Shu" points. They resemble the flow of water and are named the source points, well points, stream points, river points, and sea points.

The Five Phases

Wu Xing: Cause and Effect, the Circle is Unbroken

> *A storm in the mountains,*
> *and the valley is flooded*

The theory of the Five Phases—wood, fire, earth, metal, and water—sometimes known as the Five Elements and originally as the Five Virtues, has grown in complexity and use over the centuries. It has always been the most controversial of all the theories of Chinese medicine. This theory classifies phenomena into five quintessential categories representing phases of a continuously moving process. It holds that various phenomena existing within each phase of this cycle correspond to one another in function, quality, or other noticeable ways. For example, the phase named Wood can be seen to begin the cycle and is therefore associated with springtime, birth, and uprising. At the end of the cycle is Water, corresponding to winter, death, and hibernation.

The Five Phases also describe the relationships of the organs to each other. Like its Western counterpart, Chinese medicine recognizes that the body's organs are dependent on one another, but uses these symbolic concepts to describe their interrelation.

Each phase relates to the other according to two cycles of influence.

The first is the generating cycle (clockwise, affecting the next element). For example, the liver, overheated by anger, can attack the heart.

The second is the checking cycle (counterclockwise, skipping over the preceding phase). For example, insomnia associated with the heart-fire phase can be caused or exacerbated by a weakened kidney water phase failing to check the fire. Disharmony in one phase creates disharmony in others, according to these cycles, leading to illness.

Each phase also corresponds to a major organ system, and has a corresponding taste, color, odor, emotion, and other qualities. Some of these correspondences are:

Correspondences Associated with the Five Phases

	Wood	Fire	Earth	Metal	Water
Direction	East	South	Center	West	North
Season	Spring	Summer	Late Summer	Fall	Winter
Atmosphere	Wind	Summer Heat	Dampness	Dryness	Cold
Voice	Shout	Laugh	Sing	Weep	Groan
Color	Green	Red	Yellow	White	Black
Taste	Sour	Bitter	Sweet	Spicy	Salty
Smell	Goatlike	Burning	Fragrant	Rank	Rotten
Zhang Organ	Liver	Heart	Spleen	Lungs	Kidneys
Fu Organ	Gallbladder	Small Intestine	Stomach	Large Intestine	Bladder
Portal	Eyes	Tongue	Mouth	Nose	Ears
Body Tissue	Sinews	Blood Vessels	Flesh	Skin/Hair	Bones
Feeling	Anger	Happiness	Pensiveness	Sadness	Fear

When using the framework of the Five Phases, the practitioner examines aspects of a patient's appearance or demeanor that may implicate an organ system by virtue of correspondences. Once the organs are isolated, the known cycles of influence allow the practitioner to understand the likely root of the disease as well as its potential course. For example, a patient complaining of fatigue is observed to have black circles under her eyes. Because black alludes to the kidneys, the practitioner suspects kidney deficiency. The kidney cycles next to the liver and is considered a mother to the liver. Liver-related symptoms such as headaches, depression, or joint pain are therefore anticipated.

Occasionally, a patient with some Chinese medicine experience asks which "type" they are. They may have read Harriet Beinfield and Efrem Korngold's wonderful book, *Between Heaven and Earth*, or heard of using the theory of the Five Phases as a tool for self-awareness. This practice assumes that each person is born into one of these five types. In this self-help book, understanding the nature of one's type can further the understanding of oneself and others. For those interested in this point of view, I direct them to this seminal work.

My view is a little different. I see all theories of Traditional Chinese Medicine as subordinate to the single idea of change, which affects everything at every level. Understanding change is paramount in keeping or restoring lost balance. Views provided by theories such as the Five Phases are most valuable as pictures snapped in the flow of time. Though likely much can be gained by typing oneself, the actual practice is contrary to learning about change. Are people better off seeing themselves as fixed prototypes, always subject to the same influences and predictably inclined to the same actions? Or are they better off with a vision of themselves as free of such fixed destinies, as capable of changing and moving from phase to phase as the innumerable forces of life dictate? I believe the latter. But whatever one believes, the efficacy of Chinese medicine remains.

The Five Emotions

The five emotions transform into fire
Chinese Medicine Precept

The mind matters. In the view of Chinese medicine practitioners, emotions are a common cause of disease. The mind reaches every cell of the body, so mind and body are not distinct from one another. Paranoia and schizophrenia, like arthritis or a headache, can thus arise from physical or emotional events.

The health consequences of feelings, emotions, thoughts, and other aspects of the mind are well understood by traditional Chinese medicine. Joy, sadness, grief, fear, and anger make up the Five Emotions of Chinese philosophy, each of which relates to one of the five internal organs as described above in the Five Phases. Events in the mind affect the body chemistry. Adrenalin, epinephrine, endorphins, and thousands of chemicals are being produced, used, and disposed of at any given moment. Thoughts sweep through the body, creating a wake of altered chemistry. This changing inner chemistry influences Qi, the organs, and the rhythm of the body.

We sense these changes as "our feelings." People can sense the state of the body's inner chemistry through feelings and emotions. When feelings are intense, they warn that health can be altered in profound ways. Excessively strong emotions pervert the Qi to create disease. For example, excessive anger leads to the constraint of Qi, taxing the liver. This is felt as depression, stagnation, and a multitude of physical ailments. In another example, a person feeling extreme or prolonged fear drains their kidney Qi. This could have repercussions on the urinary, reproductive, or nervous systems, all of which are associated with the kidney.

According to Chinese medicine, our emotions affect our organs according to the theory of correspondences. Extremes in joy affect the heart, sadness affects the spleen, grief affects the lungs, fear affects the kidneys, and anger affects the liver. In reality, feelings can be difficult to clearly define. Fear and anger can intermingle with grief. The effects of emotions do not always follow a predictable path.

Feelings, and the emotions projected from them, represent the "feel" of the body's inner chemistry, or the sense of an inner landscape, and are meant for guidance.

The Twelve Organs

The Zhang Fu

> "The line drawn between spirit and matter in all characteristic Chinese thinking [is] extremely vague."
> Joseph Needham, *Science and Civilization in China*, Cambridge University Press

According to the theory of Traditional Chinese Medicine, the term "organs" refers to the physical organs in the gut, which are those known to modern science. However, the Chinese believe that internal organs perform additional functions that have to do with the production, distribution, and storage of Qi in the body. Organs can be understood as a collection of those functions, similar to a physiological "system," such as the respiratory system. For example, professionals of both Western and Chinese medicine understand that the lungs extract and distribute life-giving substance from the air. Lungs protect the inner body by filtering the air, and provide further organ protection by regulating the opening and closing of the pores. Therefore, in Chinese medicine, the lungs are thought to regulate a specialized form of Qi called defensive Qi that protects the body. Therefore, treating many immune problems often requires treating the lung Qi.

To the TCM practitioner, Qi is paramount. The biological function of the organ is often considered secondary, because when Qi is normal, an organ will behave normally. Excluding cases of physical trauma, the organs should behave normally when they are properly serviced by normal flows of Qi and blood. When organs misbehave, the Qi that sustains them usually must be regulated. Organ problems can result from Blocked Qi, Excess Qi, Vacuous Qi, Abnormal Qi, Perverse Qi, or Evil Qi. After diagnosing the underlying cause of an organ's distress, acupuncture and herbs can be administered appropriately.

Chinese medical theory groups the organs into six yin and yang pairs:

The Yin Organs are the heart, spleen, lungs, kidneys, liver, and pericardium (surface of the heart). They are called the "Zhang" (means solid) and are considered the most important. They are responsible for the regulation and storage of Qi and blood.

The Yang Organs are the stomach, small intestine, large intestine, urinary bladder, gallbladder, and triple-warmer (a functional conglomerate of all the yang organs). They are known as the "Fu" (means hollow) and are considered less important. They are responsible mainly for transportation, digestion, and elimination. The sixth pair of organs, known as the Pericardium and Triple-Heater, has energetic functions not attributed to the other organs.

Organ Pairs	Yang Functions
Heart Small Intestine	Circulates blood Transports food and fluids
Spleen Stomach	Extracts energy from food Regulates the muscles
Lung Large Intestine	Circulates Qi Regulates the surface Regulates conveyance
Kidney Urinary Bladder	Regulates urination and reproduction, nourishes brain and marrow Controls the fire at the Gate of Life
Liver Gallbladder	Smoothes the flow of Qi Regulates menstrual flow

The Gate of Life, also known as the *ming men*, is an acupuncture point located on the spine between the second and third lumbar vertebrae opposite the navel. It is called the Gate of Life because it is the center of Prenatal Qi or innate life force. Traditionally, it is considered the root of one's nature and the sea of essence and blood. This point is thought to influence transformation and generation, and is called the "mother of the spleen and stomach" and the "hole of life and death."

The Twelve Organs system's esoteric concepts do not lend themselves to scientific scrutiny. They lack the exactness and detail seen in Western medical literature. However, they help practitioners of Traditional Chinese Medicine reflect on the causes of ailments and choose the appropriate customized treatment for each patient. Meditating on or examining these ideas furthers understanding. Chinese medicine draws its value from its ability to generalize and perceive patterns that are invisible to others.

		Yin Functions
		Home to the shen (spirit) Governs blood, speech, and vessels
		Governs transportation and transformation Root of construction and the blood
		Protects the interior Governs Qi, root of Qi Governs skin and hair Stores the po (aspect of spirit)
		Stores the original Qi (yuan Qi) Stores the essence (jing) Rules the bones, brain, and marrow
		Cleans toxins Governs coursing, discharge, and movement. Stores the blood. Home to the hun (aspect of spirit)

Applying the Theories

Theories are fun like games are fun. But to be useful, they must also be instructive and true. Theories of Chinese medicine are maps of nature. Practitioners use these maps to better understand nature, including the nature of a disharmony. If these theories are accurate, they provide insight into how natural laws work and, hopefully, into the source, cause, course, and healing of ailments.

Theories are not just for practitioners and professionals. Everyone has the ability and the right to use theories. Patients use them to gain insight about the optimal care of their bodies. Seeing life in terms of yin and yang can be enlightening, helping to reveal extremes, patterns, and behaviors that cause harm.

Practitioners use these theories in markedly different ways. Some Chinese practitioners favor a particular theory and use it as a lens to view all their patients. For example, a "Five Phases practitioner" will use this theory, exclusive of all others, to select acupuncture points or herbs.

Others prefer to suit the theory to the situation. When I view pain- and injury-related problems and discuss them with patients or other practitioners, I rely on the theory of "The Channels" and of "Qi and Blood" circulation. However, I find that disharmonies stemming from emotional sources are better understood through theories of the Five Emotions or Five Phases.

Despite its many theories, Chinese medicine remains an empirical and practical medicine, its remedies and effectiveness drawn from thousands of years of practical application. Trial, error, and experience chart the treatment plan much more often than does theory.

Therefore, you can get practical results from this book regardless of how well you understand the principles in this chapter. Find your ailment in the succeeding chapters and simply follow the instructions.

4

Chinese Medicine in Action: Case Studies

The great doctor John H. Shen always reminded his students, "Disease is rooted in the life of the patient." Thus, the correct diagnosis is based on understanding the life of the patient. It is not limited to immediate symptoms. Each practitioner may assess the patient differently and come to dissimilar conclusions. Just as many roads lead to a destination, varied Chinese medicine approaches may lead to the same resolution to the "disease."

Diagnosing Olga

The following case study is an example of how my particular diagnostic process works, drawing from several theories and weaving them together to form a diagnosis. I do not claim that my method is superior to that of other professionals. Rather, it shows how I think in my daily practice, and provides a glimpse of how Chinese medicine practitioners process patient information.

Olga, a single, forty-five-year-old preschool teacher, came for relief of insomnia and fatigue. Questioning revealed that she had more trouble staying asleep than falling asleep, and when she awakened, she noticed feeling warm. She often felt irritable, and was short-tempered with her coworkers and the children in her care. She attributed this to lack of sleep. Her gynecologist had diagnosed early menopause and had prescribed hormone therapy.

During our consultation, she revealed that she was often thirsty, and felt exhausted each morning, even on the rare occasions when she slept well. She also complained of occasional lower back pain that had persisted over many years. She emitted a distinctly sour odor, had a gray-green facial tone, and flushed while speaking. Her voice was monotone. Her tongue tip was red, the tongue body pale, and the coating slightly greenish. Her pulse felt fast and weak, especially in the kidney position, where it was very deep, requiring strong pressure to feel it.

My most vivid observation was the sour odor and the green tint of her complexion and tongue; I therefore suspected a disharmony of the wood element, which corresponds to the color green as well as to the liver organ. Treating the liver was obvious, but the question was how. There are many different Chinese medicine treatments for the liver. Using common terminology, practitioners can sooth the liver, dredge the liver, nourish the liver, or cool the liver. The exact nature of the treatment is discerned by looking deeper. The theory of Five Phases helps explain the nature of the distress. According to these principles, the kidney is mother to the liver, preceding it in the generating cycle. When the liver is in distress, look first at the kidney as the source. Noting Olga's chronic lower back pain and deep kidney pulse, I diagnosed the kidney as the likely source of disharmony, and realized it must be adjusted before an effective treatment of the liver would work.

According to the Five Phases theory, wood generates fire; therefore, the liver is mother to the heart. It also predicts that heart-related symptoms could appear if the liver is out of balance. In Olga's case, this had already happened, judging by her insomnia, irritability, and red-tipped tongue.

My treatment plan started to take shape. I knew that it must encompass at least three elements: water (kidney), wood (liver), and fire (heart). I knew with certainty that I must assist Olga to restore harmony, balance, and normalcy to these three organs. Whatever the nature of the distress, normalcy is the cure. Body imbalances, no matter how chemically complex, can be expressed symbolically as yin and yang. The theory of yin and yang illuminates the nature of this imbalance. Restoring balance depends on discerning yin from yang and knowing which is in excess and which is deficient. When yin and yang are in proper balance, normalcy follows. All Chinese medicine practitioners evaluate their patients in terms of yin and yang, doing their best to determine what is in excess and what is deficient. Once this is completed, a treatment plan is apparent. This evaluation is based on what stands out or is prominent in the appearance, demeanor, behavior, and history of the individual.

The Theory of the Organs reveals that the kidney is a great repository of Qi. Surplus Qi is stored there. Olga's weak lower back and fatigue indicate a deficiency of kidney energy. Her thirst, dry skin, and heat-disturbed sleep pointed to a deficiency of yin fluids. It appeared that Olga's kidney yin, which would normally generate her liver yin fluids and in turn cool her liver, had become deficient, thus failing to cool the liver sufficiently, causing the liver yang to heat up, rising to scorch the heart, resulting in symptoms of rapid pulse, insomnia, and irritability.

In Chinese medicine terminology, my working diagnosis was "deficient kidney yin generates deficient liver yin causing excess yang of the liver and heart." My treatment plan became clear. To restore balance, I needed to assist Olga to strengthen the deficient yin fluids of both her liver and kidney and to reduce the excess yang fire in her liver and heart.

Armed with a working diagnosis, I then developed a treatment strategy. Having a plan provides perspective, guidance, and focus. Such a plan should prognosticate the length of time needed for symptomatic relief as well as complete resolution. The treatment plan should evaluate all available options, such as massage, movement, meditation, particular acupuncture points, and specific herbal formulas.

Since Olga had experienced sleep problems for five years, I anticipated approximately five months of treatment to affect a cure. But many of my patients feel better within days. I find most people with insomnia experience some relief after one or two acupuncture treatments or within a week of taking herbs.

I planned to put Olga on an acupuncture and herb regimen, but first suggested something else. From her voice, I suspected she felt dulled or depressed, so I recommended that she try to add something new to her life. As she reclined on her back on the acupuncture table, we discussed Tai Chi, yoga, and writing classes. But after I tapped a small needle in her third-eye point, *yintang*, her body relaxed and her eyes closed. I placed thin needles in the insides of her wrists in the heart and pericardium channels. Endorphins seeped like morphine into her bloodstream; soon she was asleep.

After thirty minutes, Olga woke up, forgetting at first where she was. I jokingly congratulated her on surviving her first acupuncture treatment. She said it was the best sleep she had experienced in years. I described her first herbal prescription, a combination of two popular formulas: *shui de an*, known for its ability to calm the spirit and clear heat from the heart, plus *zhi bai di huang*, to strengthen yin, and nourish the body's cooling and lubricating fluids.

Olga was a practitioner's dream, a rare model patient who responds to all treatments by the book. After about six months of herbs and acupuncture, she was fundamentally cured. I see her now and then for minor ailments, but not for chronic insomnia or fatigue.

I wish all my patients were like Olga, but I must claim: "Your mileage may vary." Most people experience noticeable relief, and acute, simple problems are often resolved immediately. Difficult problems are usually difficult for everybody, including practitioners of Traditional Chinese Medicine.

Mr. Brown and Mr. Silver

Same Disease, Different Medicines

Chinese medical practitioners are fond of saying, "We treat the patient, not the disease." The treatment plan must fit the whole patient, including the patient's complaints, unique constitution, as well as the environmental, atmospheric, or emotional circumstances that may influence his or her condition. Therefore, two people who have been diagnosed with the same disease may receive different treatments and advice. Mr. Brown and Mr. Silver are two such cases.

Mr. Brown and Mr. Silver both came to see me in 2002. Both were in their early thirties, overweight, complained of knee pain, and suffered from tendonitis of the same tendons. Both had been prescribed the same pain medicines by their MD physicians.

From my vantage point, the differences between these two young men were at least as important as the similarities. Both received acupuncture at the same points, but the rest of their respective treatment plans was different due to their individual profiles.

Brown was an athlete and Silver was a teacher. Brown was a celebrated offensive lineman for the Oakland Raiders. He came once a week during one football season. Though his massive torso never showed obvious signs of injury or bruising, he suffered about a hundred aches and pains, including the knee pain under treatment.

His medical diagnosis of tendonitis was appropriate, but had little relevance to me. The relevant point was that his tendonitis stemmed from physical trauma and repeated stress. He was literally getting beaten up each week.

Brown was otherwise healthy. His pulse was strong. His tongue was normal, and he revealed no other complaints. Because of all these circumstances, his diagnosis was Blood and Qi Stagnation due to first-, second-, and third-stage injuries. I developed a treatment plan to help him survive his weekly assaults so he could keep playing football.

I gave him electro-acupuncture on points on and near the knee as well as points located distal to the knee on the same ankle, Ching

Koo pills for injury, and Tieh Ta Yao Gin ointment to apply topically. At first, I reluctantly concurred with his trainer's advice to ice the knee to reduce swelling and pain and allow him to continue playing. But I warned Brown that using ice could produce a long-term detrimental effect.

In contrast, Silver's knee injury was a mystery to him; he remembered hurting it many years ago as a teenager, but could not remember injuring it in the recent past. He just woke up one day and it hurt. X-rays showed no fractures, dislocations, or arthritis. Without evidence of any other known condition, he, too, had been diagnosed with tendonitis.

From the perspective of Chinese medicine, however, Silver was very different from Brown. Questioning revealed that he had several other complaints. He caught colds easily and often felt tired. The quality of his pain was different from Brown's, which was sharp and stabbing with movement but disappeared when his leg was resting. Silver described his pain as deep and throbbing, severe with movement, but nevertheless still achy when at rest. His pulse was weak, and his tongue was pale. When the damp San Francisco Bay Area fog rolled in, Silver's knee got worse while Brown's did not.

Silver's tendonitis was related to a deficiency rather than to a recent injury. My diagnosis was Damp Bi Syndrome caused by vacuity of *wei Qi*. In English, it means that the energy that normally helps to protect the knee from the outer environment had weakened. This allowed atmospheric damp to penetrate the surface of the body, impairing flow in the joints and tendons, a very common condition, but still a mystery to modern medicine. This knee was particularly vulnerable because its Qi had been weakened by the earlier injury.

Silver was given acupuncture at almost the same points as Brown. However, I also treated Silver with moxibustion (heat treatment) at the same points. I prescribed Du Huo Ji Shen Wan tablets to expel damp and increase circulation in the lower body. I also gave him Zheng Gu Shui liniment to apply topically. I told him to ignore his doctor's advice and to avoid using ice under any circumstance. Because his condition was susceptible to damp invasion, I also told him not to soak the knee or to use wet compresses of any kind.

Both patients fared fairly well during treatment, but Brown's case was an uphill battle week to week. I knew that he was keenly aware of the toll football was taking on his body. Though I never saw him after that season, I heard he retired two years later.

After a handful of acupuncture treatments that were not miraculous, I also lost track of Silver as a patient. But something must have helped; he still comes by our shop regularly to buy Zheng Gu Shui liniment.

John, Rita, and Patrick

Same Medicine, Different Diseases

It is not unusual for different patients suffering unrelated maladies to receive the exact same medicine. There are several reasons for this. The most obvious is that underlying imbalances can manifest in different ways, producing differing symptoms and complaints. These manifestations receive different modern medical diagnosis. Another reason has to do with the complexity of these formulas and the evolving experience in their use. Some of these formulas have been in daily use for thousands of years. During that time, practitioners learned how to use them to satisfy different medical strategies. Take the case of *jin gui shen qi wan*, also described in Chapter 5, "Famous Herbal Medicines."

John was fifty-five years old and had just remarried. He was in excellent physical condition, worked out at a gym several times a week, and was a near vegetarian. He had only one complaint. He reported that for the last few months it had become difficult for him to obtain and sustain an erection, and he was reluctant to use prescribed drugs as he feared their side effects. With difficulty, he was able to ejaculate, but the ejaculations were weak and unsatisfying. Furthermore, ejaculation produced a feeling of total exhaustion and soreness in his lower back.

Though a robust and imposing-looking man, his pulse was extremely deep and difficult to feel in the kidney position on both wrists. His tongue was normal except for a small bald patch deep toward the root of the tongue. When I asked about the frequency of his ejaculations, he answered that he and his new (and much younger) bride were trying to have a baby, and so were having sex daily, sometimes twice a day.

John's diagnosis was Deficiency of Kidney Qi. Sexual gymnastics appropriate for a teenager will quickly deplete a middle-aged man. My advice to John was to reduce the frequency of his ejaculations to once every five or six days. If he wanted to be potent at the right moment, he would have to conserve it. Without conservation, kidney Qi would continue to deplete faster than it could be restored. In other words, fix the leak before filling the vessel. To fill the vessel and strengthen John's erection's, the strategy was to build kidney Qi. I told him to eat an occasional hamburger (meat is considered to strengthen the kidneys), and for his erectile dysfunction, I prescribed *jin gui shen qi wan*. Though it will not work instantly, like Viagra, this formula will gradually bolster his reproductive system and probably boost his sex drive as well.

Rita was a young woman who felt old. At thirty-five, she was habitually tired, even after a good night's sleep. She often felt cold. Her hair was falling out. Her pulse felt weak and thin, like a thread, but her tongue coloring was pink and normal. She had been diagnosed as hypothyroid, deficient in thyroid hormone, by her MD doctor, who had prescribed thyroid medication. Rita wanted to know if there were any herbs that would help.

Rita's diagnosis was the same as John's: Deficiency of Kidney Qi. However, in her case, her thyroid gland, not her reproductive system, was suffering most of the effects of deficient kidney Qi. I advised her to try the herbs before taking the thyroid drugs. The prescribed thyroid medicine would likely have solved most of her complaints, but would have led to a lifelong addiction. Moreover, these drugs would not have solved the kidney Qi deficiency that was causing her poor thyroid performance, which could emerge later in life as another inexplicable pathology. If the herbs worked, they might do more than just relieve her symptoms. For my prescription for her hypothyroid condition, I added seaweed to *jin gui shen qi wan* herbs.

Patrick's chief complaint was frequent urination, which had plagued him for more than a decade. At sixty-five years old, Patrick got regular exercise and felt healthy. He did have high blood pressure and high cholesterol, both regulated by pharmaceuticals. His urologist diagnosed an enlarged prostate and gave him a prescription. Patrick was already seeing me for acupuncture for an intractable foot pain. It was simple to add a few acupuncture points—like Kidney 3 on his inner ankles, and Conception Vessel 6 below his navel—to tonify his kidney Qi. His herbal prescription for enlarged prostate was *jin gui shen qi wan*.

The diverse ailments of John, Rita, and Patrick show that *jin gui shen qi wan* is useful for a wide range of ailments. According to *Chinese Herbal Medicine Formulas and Strategies*, the most authoritative source on the use of herbal medicines, *jin gui shen qi wan* may be used in treating such disorders as chronic glomerular, interstitial or diffuse nephritis, chronic urethritis, diabetes mellitus, hypothyroidism, primary hyperaldosteronism, neurasthenia, arthritis, beriberi, and chronic bronchial asthma.

These cases illustrate how Traditional Chinese Medicine differs from Western medicine in everyday practice. I hope they reveal that each system has its own logic, and that practitioners of the two do not always draw the same conclusions because they pay attention to entirely different matters. I hope you now understand the basic concepts of yin and yang, and are fascinated about how and why Chinese medicine works. The way practitioners sense what's going on with the patient, how the patient senses the disease, and the common sense and logic of nature all guide the practice of Chinese medicine.

5

Famous Herbal Medicines

In the West, we are used to thinking that the more concentrated a medicine is, the more profound its effect. Pharmaceutical researchers, who begin with an herbal substance, eliminate as many "extraneous" chemical compounds as possible from the herb so that only the "active ingredients" remain.

The Value of Combining Herbs

Chinese medicine practitioners take a different approach. They believe that a medicine often becomes more powerful or useful by including more compounds, rather than excluding them. The Chinese learned long ago to combine herbs into complex medicines that were more powerful because of their synergy and complexity. For example, honeysuckle flowers have heat-clearing (anti-inflammatory) properties. Used alone, they have a mild and barely noticeable effect. But when combined with forsythia, the heat-clearing action is noticeably stronger than with either herb taken alone. When this blend is further combined with other heat-clearing herbs, such as chrysanthemum, phragmites, and isatides, numerous medicines with startlingly incontrovertible effects are created. Legendary Chinese cold medicines such as *yin chiao, zhong gan ling,* and *gan mao ling* are all combinations of these heat-clearing herbs

Herbs are also combined to reduce side effects. *Dang gui* is a wonderful herb for building the blood. Used in many formulas and over many centuries, it has helped provide Chinese women with good menstrual health. Taken alone, however, it can also provide annoying and unhealthy diarrhea. Therefore, unless one is constipated, it's best to combine *dang gui* with other herbs, such as Astragalus, Atractylodes, or licorice, to curb this effect.

How Formulas Are Created

Chinese doctors learned to create potent medicines from herbs long ago, and developed elaborate diagnostic theories to explain the patterns they were observing.

Regardless of theory, Chinese medicine is first and foremost practical. It has survived thousands of years because it works, not because "water quenches fire." In an empirical system such as Chinese medicine, rules exist, but they may be altered by further inquiry or discovery. There is a rule for creating herbal formulas. However, there are also countless formulas that do not appear to follow these rules. Yet they work.

Formulas usually consist of principal herbs, supporting herbs, adjuvant herbs (used to combat the side effects of other herbs), and messenger herbs.

Principal herbs must be chosen to carry out a strategy to overcome the disharmony. Heat must be cooled, dampness dried, toxins cleaned, excess drained, weakness strengthened, and so on.

Supporting herbs help the principal herbs. They also account for varying characteristics unique and appropriate to the patient and the moment.

Adjuvant herbs balance and harmonize the formula by smoothing the roughness of certain herbs, and by making the herbs more digestible and easy to assimilate.

Messenger herbs are used to direct the formula action to a specific part of the body, or to move the Qi in a specific direction.

Famous Formulas

Chinese herbal pharmacies abound with medical treasures that have been perfected by trial and error over centuries of practical use. The following medicines are among the oldest and most popular in the annals of Chinese medicine, as useful and timely now as they have ever been. Adopting these medicines into the Western medical culture can improve overall heath care. I have chosen these formulas from thousands for several reasons. They are safe for everyone. They will not cause harm if mis-prescribed. They easily outperform their pharmaceutical counterparts. Their effects are reliable and easily noticed within a relatively short time. When they are incorporated into the Western culture, they will save or improve many lives. Remember that 200,000 people die in the United States each year from non-prescribed, over-the-counter medicines.

Yin Chiao Chieh Tu Pien

Yin Chiao, Honeysuckle, and Forsythia Clean Toxin Pill

Many say that *yin chiao* is the long-sought cure for the common cold. It is 100 percent herbal, 100 percent safe, and one of nature's great gifts. Although it has been used successfully for hundreds of years, the Western world is just now catching on. The popular cold remedy Airborne® is based on the principal herbs in *yin chiao*. Airborne is essentially *yin chiao* made fizzy with added zinc and some extraneous vitamins. When Oprah Winfrey discovered that it worked, everyone took notice. Perhaps someday she will try the original formula. It works even better. This formula is used for conditions such as the common cold, influenza, upper respiratory infection, measles, swollen glands, and sore throat.

Traditional Use Use at the first sign of or during the first two days of cold or flu, and when exposed or likely to be exposed to cold or flu.

Formula Function in Chinese Medicine Terms *Yin chiao* disperses wind heat, clears heat, and relieves toxicity.

Source The yin chiao formula was first published in 1798 in Dr. Wu Ju Tong's *Wen Bing Tao Bian* (Systematic Differentiation of Warm Diseases). At the time of its publication, *yin chiao* had been in use for hundreds of years.

Dosage *Yin chiao* is taken as a tablet or powder rather than as a boiled decoction to preserve the chemical integrity of the principal herbs.

Adults: At the first sign of cold or flu, take three to five grams immediately (usually six to eight pills, depending on the brand of *yin chiao* used), then take two to three grams every four hours for the rest of the day. For prevention, take two grams (three to four tablets) every four hours when exposed to cold or flu. This formula is considered safe for pregnancy.

Children: Use 700 milligrams (usually one tablet) for each twenty-five pounds of body weight. Crush and mix with food.

Course of Use The course of treatment is a minimum of one day and a maximum of one week per episode. Bedrest during the hours of administration, when possible, is a plus.

Suggestions Keep a dozen *yin chiao* tablets in your car, purse, or pocket during cold and flu season. Take promptly when you feel a cold coming on. Begin taking tablets a half hour before entering airports, airplanes, terminals, or crowded public facilities.

Ingredients and Chinese Medicine Functions

- Honeysuckle (*jin yin hua, Lonicera flos*): clears heat, cleans toxins, and expels externally contracted wind heat.
- Forsythia (*lian Qiao, Forsythia suspensa fructus*): expels contracted wind heat, clears heat, and cleans toxins.
- Balloon flower (*jie geng, Platycodi grandiflori radix*): transforms cold phlegm, circulates lung energy, benefits the throat, and directs the action of other herbs upward.

- Peppermint (*bo he, Menthe herba*): disperses wind heat, clears the head and eyes, and benefits the throat.
- Edible burdock (*niu bang zi, Arctium lappa*): detoxifies fire poison, disperses wind heat, and benefits the throat.
- Crested grass (*dan zhu ye, Lophatheri gracilis*): releases the exterior, disperses wind heat, lessens irritability, and relieves thirst.
- Schizonepeta (*jing jie, Schizonepeta tenuifolia*): releases the exterior, and expels wind cold and wind heat.
- Fermented soy bean (*dan dou chi, Sojae praeparatum semen*): releases the exterior for both cold and hot exterior conditions, and alleviates irritability.
- Chinese licorice root (*gan cao, Glycyrrhiza uranelsis radix*): tonifies the spleen, benefits the Qi, detoxifies fire poisons, and moderates and harmonizes other herbs.

Notes   Although *yin chiao* is considered a wind heat formula, it is traditionally used and is effective for both wind heat and wind cold patterns. More reliable than other formulas used for wind cold maladies, *yin chiao* is suitable for patients who present with dryness due to deficiency of blood, or yin due to the mild and non-drying nature of the herbs used in this formula. The formula is generally considered safe during pregnancy and nursing.

Hsiao Yao San

> Other Names: *Free and Easy, Relaxed Wanderer, Rambling Powder,* and *Xiao Yao San*

Several of my teachers believe that this formula is one of the greatest gifts Chinese medicine has bestowed upon the West. *Hsiao yao san* addresses problems created by stress, so prevalent in the Western lifestyle. This condition results in modern medical diagnoses of depression, anxiety, and several kinds of psychosis, as well as many physical ailments baffling to modern medicine.

Hsiao yao san was first described in the *Imperial Grace Formulary* of the Tai Ping era (1078–1085 AD). It is commonly used to relieve depression and the constraining effects of stress on the body. Though this formula usually takes weeks or months of regular use to begin working, some people feel its effects within days.

Traditional Use When under stress, Qi (energy) tightens the chest. This protective reaction is triggered by current or remembered events. *Hsiao yao wan* reduces feelings of stress by helping to release tension in the chest. Based on a 900-year-old formula, it uses natural substances to relieve chest constraint and to promote the free flow of Qi in the chest.

The chief herb in *hsiao yao san* is Bupleurum (*chai hu*) with a small amount of mint. This combination powerfully spreads the Qi of the chest (liver Qi), relieving emotional constraint, depression, and pre-menstrual syndrome. It also helps increase the nourishing and cleansing flows of Qi and blood to the breasts, as well as to the upper and middle organs.

Other herbs in the formula, such as *Angelica sinensis* (*dang gui*) and white peony (*bai shao*), build deficient liver blood, a condition that commonly contributes to stuck Qi. The rest of the formula (licorice, ginger, Atractylodes) aids digestion and increases formula absorption.

Popular variations include *jia wei xiao yao wan*, which adds herbs to clear heat in the heart, a condition that often results from stagnation of Qi in the chest, and *long gu muli xiao yao wan*, which adds calcium-rich fossil bone and oyster shell to settle the spirit.

Hsiao yao san can also be used with other herbs or formulas when stress is an aggravating factor: stress-induced headache, stress-related digestive ills, pain below the ribs, allergies, hypertension, or any other condition made worse by stress. The formula is generally considered safe during pregnancy or nursing.

Formula Function in Chinese Medicine Terms Spreads liver Qi, builds liver blood.

Source *Imperial Grace Formulary* of the Tai Ping Era (1078–1085 AD).

Dosage Originally prescribed as a powder, *hsiao yao san* can also be taken as a pill or boiled decoction. Alcohol extracts (tinctures), however, are not recommended due to the irritating effect of alcohol on the liver. Taken as a pill or powder, the dose is three to six grams per day (about one-ninth to one-fifth of an ounce). Taken as a boiled decoction, the dose is fifteen to thirty grams per day (about one-half to one ounce per day). To make a boiled extraction from dried herbs, use about five times as much as in powder or pill form.

Course of Use   One week minimum. *Hsiao yao san* is considered safe for daily regular use as well as for pregnancy. Some women use this formula during the later part of their menstrual cycle, from ovulation until the onset of menses, to prevent or relieve premenstrual syndrome (PMS).

Suggestions   *Hsiao yao san* is most effective when used together with a program of physical activity to relieve stress and constraint in the upper body.

Ingredients and Chinese Medicine Functions
* Hare's ear root (*chai hu, Bupleurum chinense*): relaxes constrained Qi, and releases exterior.
* White peony root (*bai shao, Paeonia*): pacifies the liver and nourishes the blood.
* *Tang gui* root (*dang gui, Angelica sinensis*): harmonizes and tonifies the blood.
* Hoelin (*fu ling, Poria cocos sclerotum*): quiets the heart, calms the spirit, harmonizes the middle, and strengthens the spleen.
* White Atractylodes (*bai zhu, Atractylodes*): benefits the Qi, stabilizes the exterior, strengthens the spleen, and dries dampness.
* Ginger (*sheng jiang, Zinzeberis*): releases the exterior, disperses cold, and adjusts the nutritive and protective.
* Chinese licorice root (*gan cao, Glycyrrhizae*): harmonizes other herbs, clears heat, detoxifies fire poison, and benefits the Qi.
* Mint leaf (*bo he, Mentha folium*): frees constrained Qi, clears the head and eyes, and disperses wind heat.

Notes   The effectiveness of *hsiao yao san* can be heightened by increasing the proportion of *Bupleurum chinense* (*chai hu*) in the formula. This is the principal herb for activating the Qi of the chest. One can also add herbs that have a similar function, such as mimosa bark (*he huan pi*) or flowers (*he huan hua*).

Ba Zhen Wan

Other Names: *Eight Treasures, Women's Precious Pills*

Ba zhen wan is used for menstrual good health and to benefit the body's nourishing flows of blood (nourishment) and Qi (energy). When blood and Qi are weak, the body goes hungry regardless of diet. Woman's Precious Pill is used as a daily supplement to boost and maintain blood and Qi. Though both men and women use the pill, most often women use it to supplement regular blood loss due to menstruation. It is especially useful for women who eat little or no red meat. This formula is considered safe to take throughout pregnancy and nursing. It is often used in cases of infertility, when blood deficiency is a contributing factor. It is appropriate in all cases of anemia. We find that it works a lot better than iron supplements for this purpose.

Traditional Uses Treating blood and Qi deficiency caused by spleen deficiency.

Functions in Chinese Medicine Terms *Ba zhen wan* strengthens the blood, Qi, and spleen

Source The *Ba zhen wan* formula was first published in the *Zheng Ti Lei Yao* (Catalogued Essentials for Correcting the Body) by Dr. Bi Lai Zhai in the year 1529.

Dosage Taken as a pill or powder, three to six grams are recommended daily for health maintenance. Relieving symptoms can require up to ten grams daily. Ideally, these are taken in three doses, preferably on an empty stomach. It may be easier to take *ba zhen wan* twice a day, half in the morning and half in the evening. For boiled decoctions, use five times as much.

Course of Use The course of use is a minimum of one month and a maximum of eleven months per year. We recommend occasionally resting from all long-term formulas. Women's Precious Pill can be taken with *ba zhen wan* to help ease post-partum depression.

Suggestions As with most strengthening-oriented Chinese herbal tonics, discontinue use during cold and flu.

Ingredients and Functions

*   *Dang gui,* Chinese angelica root (*tang kwei, dong guai, Angelica sinensis radix*): strengthens blood, invigorates blood, harmonizes blood, and regulates menses.
*   White peony root (*bai shao, Peonia lactiflora*): nourishes the blood, pacifies the liver, and retains the yin.
*   Chinese foxglove root (*shu di huang, Rehmannia glutinosa*): tonifies the blood, and tonifies the heart, liver, and kidneys.
*   Szechuan lovage root (*chuan xiong, Liguistici wallichi*): invigorates the blood, promotes the circulation of Qi (energy), and expels wind.
*   Poor man's ginseng (*dang shen, Codonopsis radix*): benefits the Qi, nourishes fluids, and strengthens the lungs and digestive organs.
*   *Bai zhu* (*Atractylodes macrocephala rhizome*): benefits the Qi, tonifies the spleen, and dries dampness.
*   *Fu ling* (*Poria cocos sclerotum* or Hoelen fungus): leeches out dampness, strengthens digestion, harmonizes the middle burner, calms the spirit, and improves the performance of other tonifying herbs.
*   Chinese licorice root baked with honey (*zhi gan cao, Glycyrrhiza uranelsis radix*): tonifies the spleen, benefits the Qi, detoxifies fire poisons, moderates and harmonizes other herbs, and improves the performance of other tonifying herbs.

Notes The herb *Angelica sinensis* (*dang gui*) should not be administered as a single herb. It is always combined with other herbs. The blend used in Woman's Precious Pill is the most widely used of these combinations. It brings out the best qualities of the herb while eliminating unwanted side effects. Though this formula is used as a daily supplement to maintain good health, it is also used to treat symptoms related to deficiencies, such as fatigue, weakness, menstrual irregularities, tired limbs, pallor, pale tongue, infertility, shortness of breath or palpitations, lightheadedness, and reduced appetite.

Most modern versions of this formula use *dang shen* (Codonopsis) instead of *ren shen* (ginseng), making it more cost effective and more tonifying to the spleen, thus helping to better assimilate the four blood tonic herbs.

Ko Ning Wan

Stomach Curing Pills, Po Chai Pills

Not a traditional formula, this patent medicine evolved from Preserve Harmony Pill (*bao he wan*) which first appeared in *The Teachings of Zhu* by Zhu Zheng Heng, 1481. This herbal wonder relieves nausea and/or headache due to stomach flu, overeating, hangover, unfamiliar diet, motion sickness, morning sickness, simple indigestion, and the like. Curing pills, *ko ning wan*, are a fixture in every Chinese medicine cabinet, and a must for world travelers.

Traditional Uses   Nausea, vomiting, mild food poisoning, hangover, indigestion, stomach flu, belching

Formula Function in Chinese Medicine Terms   *Ko ning wan* (Stomach Curing Pill) reduces food stagnation, sends rebellious stomach Qi downwards, clears heat, dries dampness

Source   Preserve Harmony Pill (*Bao He Wan*). *Teachings of Zhu* (1481 AD).

Dosage   *Ko ning wan* is best taken as a pill or powder to avoid drinking a large amount of liquid when nauseous. Taken as a pill or powder, three to six grams as needed usually works within twenty minutes.

Ingredients
- Costus root (*mu xiang, Saussureae radix*): moves the Qi, dissipates stagnant intestinal Qi, and alleviates pain.

- Angelica root (*bai zhi, Angelica dahurica*): expels wind, releases surface, alleviates pain, reduces swelling, expels dampness, and alleviates discharge.
- Medicated leaven (*shen qu, Massa fermentata*): dissolves food, transforms accumulations, and aides digestion.
- Mint leaf (*bo he, Mentha folium*): frees constrained Qi, clears the head and eyes, and disperses wind heat.
- Citrus peel (*chen pi, Citri rubrum exocarpum*): moves the Qi, strengthens spleen, dries dampness, directs the Qi downward, and prevents stagnation.
- Chrysanthemum (*ju hua, Chrysanthemomi flos*): disperses wind, clears heat from the eyes, and pacifies the liver.
- Ornamental orchid (*tian ma, Gastrodia rhiz*): pacifies the liver, extiguishes wind, alleviates pain, and disperses painful obstruction.
- Hoelin mushroom (*fu ling, Poria cocos*): quiets the heart, calms the spirit, harmonizes the middle, and strengthens stomach/spleen.
- Job's tears (*yi yi ren, Coicis semen*): leaches dampness, strengthens stomach/spleen, clears damp heat, and reduces diarrhea.
- Magnolia bark (*hou po, Magnolia cortex*): moves the Qi, transforms dampness, resolves stagnation, and directs rebellious Qi downward.
- Patchouli (*huo xiang, Agastach pogostemi*): transforms dampness, releases the exterior, harmonizes the center, and expels dampness.
- White Atractylodes (*bai zhu, Atractylodes*): benefits the Qi, stabilizes the exterior, strengthens the spleen, and dries dampness.
- Rice sprout (*gu ya, Oryzae germinantus*): dissolves food stagnation and strengthens stomach.
- Kudzu root (*ge gen, Pueraria radix*): clears heat, releases muscles of upper body, and nourishes fluids.

Notes This formula is meant to relieve symptoms and is for acute, short-term use. Prolonged use is not recommended and could harm digestion.

Rehmannia Combinations

Liu Wei Di Huang Rehmannia Six Combination

Zhi Bai Di Huang Rehmannia Six plus *zhi mu* and *huang bai*, also known as Rehmannia Eight Combination

Gui Fu Di Huang Rehmannia Six plus cinnamon and aconite, also known as Golden Book Pill

Ming Mu Di Huang Bright Eyes Rehmannia combination

Tian Huang Bu Xin Wan Heavenly Emperor Strengthen Heart Pill

Rehmannia (*shu si huang*) is also known as Chinese foxglove root. It is an amazing herb, unequalled in ability to strengthen the blood and yin of the liver and kidney. Like most Chinese medicine herbs, it is always used in formula and very rarely alone. These are variations of the famous kidney yin tonic *liu wei di huang*, also known as Rehmannia Six Combination. This formula is renowned for its ability to strengthen the yin of the entire body. Think of the yin as the fluids of the body. These fluids nourish, lubricate, and cool. Yin deficiencies often result in weakness, inflammation, friction, and heat. Severe forms of yin deficiency can include many chronic conditions including chronic fatigue, chronic pain, night sweats, and chronic inflammatory conditions.

Traditional Uses Treatment of adult onset diabetes, chronic fatigue, impotence, frequent urination, weakness in the lower back and knees, chronic scratchy throat or persistent flu-like symptoms, insomnia, chronic mild toothache, dry skin, cataracts, and other clinical conditions

Formula Functions in Chinese Medicine Terms Although various versions have different applications, Rehmannia combinations strengthen the yin and blood of the liver and kidney.

Source The *jin gui shen qi wan* formula, known above as Golden Book Pill, was first published in *Essentials from the Golden Cabinet* between 150 and 219 AD.

Dosage Take more to overcome symptoms. Take less for daily maintenance. Taken as a pill or powder, the dose is three to six grams per day (about one-ninth to one-fifth of an ounce). The number of pills will vary according to the size of the pill. It takes four 750 mg tablets to deliver three grams of medicine, but it takes fifteen 200 mg "teapills" to equal three grams.

Taken as a boiled decoction, the dose is fifteen to thirty grams per day (about one half to one ounce).

Course of Use One week minimum. This formula is considered safe for daily regular use as well as during pregnancy.

Suggestions Some versions of this formula are considered a bit hard to digest. If you have problems digesting any of the rehmannia combinations, try taking them with food, hawthorn berries, or ginger tea.

Ingredients and Functions The base formula is *liu wei* (six ingredients). The two variations contain the six herbs used in *liu wei*. However, *zhi bai di huang* adds *zhi mu* and *huang bai* to clear the deficiency heat that is common in yin-deficient individuals. (The names of many Chinese herbal formulas are formed this way, by combining the names of their principal ingredients.) Signs of heat deficiency include afternoon fever, night sweats, hot flashes, heat in soles of feet or palms, insomnia, restlessness, and other symptoms. People who generally feel warm and tired use this version. People who feel cold and/or have trouble digesting it should avoid *liu wei*.

Golden Book Pill (*Treasure from the Golden Cabinet*) adds *rou gui* (cinnamon bark) and *fu zi* (processed aconite root) to *liu wei di huang* to make *gui fu di huang*. This variation warms the original formula, making it appropriate for kidney yang deficiency with cold presentations, as well as for people with spleen deficiency (weak digestion) who are unable to digest other variations of Rehmannia Six. People who generally feel cold and tired use Golden Book Pills.

Notes Although Rehmannia Six is the primary formula used to strengthen the yin, not a single herb in the formula is classified as a yin tonic. The formula consists of herbs that build blood, build Qi, astringe essence, clear heat, and move water. Yet the total effect of the formula, its synergy, is to tonify the yin.

Si Jun Zi Wan Four Gentlemen

Liu Jun Zi Wan Six Gentlemen

These two are the most tried and true formulas for simple spleen deficiency (weak digestion). Spleen deficiency can manifest with symptoms of both weak Qi and weak blood. This can include poor enzyme production, slow digestion, loose or erratic stools, bloating, anemia, fatigue, or lethargy.

The "spleen" in Chinese medicine is very different than the organ you know as your spleen. Ancient practitioners did not differentiate between the spleen and pancreas. They were considered to be one. Hence, the Chinese medicine spleen includes the functions of your pancreas. It's kind of the brain of your digestive system. It influences the function of all the digestive organs. Spleen Qi deficiency can underlie many digestive problems, including diseases of the pancreas, esophagus, and large and small intestines.

Traditional Uses Persistent diarrhea, loose or erratic stool, fatigue, lethargy, muscle weakness, shortness of breath, abdominal bloating, excessive flatulence, borborygmus (stomach growling), low appetite, pale complexion, and weak voice.

Formula Functions in Chinese Medicine Terms Strengthens the spleen and regulates (moves) the spleen Qi

Source *Imperial Grace Formulary* of the Tai Ping Era (1078–1085).

Dosage Take more to overcome symptoms, less for daily maintenance. Taken as a pill or powder, the dose is three to six grams per day (about one-ninth to one-fifth of an ounce). Taken as a boiled decoction, the dose is fifteen to thirty grams per day (about one-half to one ounce per day).

Course of Use One week or longer. This formula is generally considered safe for regular use as well as for pregnancy, however overuse can cause dry mouth, thirst, or constipation.

Suggestions The version known as Four Gentlemen is considered a base formula and is almost always enhanced with other herbs. Six Gentlemen is preferable for most people.

Ingredients and Functions

The Four Gentlemen:
1. Two parts Chinese sage root (*dang shen, Codonopsis radix*)
2. Two parts Hoelen mushroom (*fu ling, Poria cocos*)
3. Two parts atractylodes root (*bai zhu, Atractylodes radix*)
4. One part licorice root baked with honey (*zhi gan cao, Glycyrrhiza radix*)

The Six Gentlemen adds two herbs:
1. Prepared pinellia rhizome (*ban xia*)
2. Citrus peel (*chen pi*)

The two make the formula more effective for damp accumulations due to weak spleen or food stagnation. This condition can result symptoms such as a persistent cough with thin or watery sputum, chronic sinus congestion, runny nose, or cough after eating. This formula can be useful for some types of morning sickness.

Er Xiang Wan Two Immortals Pill

This modern formula was originally developed for menopausal hypertension, but is often used to treat other menopausal symptoms as well as certain other forms of hypertension.

Traditional Uses Complaints associated with menopause, such as fatigue, low libido, hot flashes, high blood pressure, day or night sweats, and insomnia

Formula Function in Chinese Medicine Terms Replenish

kidney yang and yin, build blood, and clear deficiency heat.

Source   *Traditional Chinese Medical Formulas*, Shanghai College of Traditional Medicine, 1975. The name Two Immortals (*er xian*) comes from two of the chief herbs in the formula: *xian mao* (*curculigo*) and *xian ling pi* (*epemidii*).

Dosage   Take more to overcome symptoms, less for daily maintenance. Taken as a pill or powder, the dose is three to six grams per day (about one-ninth to one-fifth of an ounce). Taken as a boiled decoction, the dose is fifteen to thirty grams per day (about one-half to one ounce per day).

Course of Use   Take as a daily supplement for periods of two weeks or longer. Acceptable for long-term use, but discontinue use periodically. Rest one to three months per year, or one week per month. As with many tonic formulas, discontinue use during a cold or flu.

Suggestions   First-day results are unusual. Benefits are usually seen after one to five weeks.

As with most Chinese herbal tonics, Two Immortals Pills should not be taken while ill with cold or flu. Tonics are thought to prolong such illnesses. Wait until the cold or flu has passed before resuming course of treatment.

Ingredients and Functions
- Morinda root (*bai ji tan, Radix morinda officianalis*): tonifies the kidneys, fortifies the kidneys, fortifies the yang, and strengthens the sinews and bones.
- Licentious goat wort (*yin yang huo, Herba epimedi*): stimulates hormone production, tonifies the yin, fortifies the yang, and expels dampness.
- Golden eye grass (*xian mao, Rhizoma curculinginis orchioidis*): tonifies the kidneys and expels dampness.
- Amur cork bark (*huang bai, Cortex phellodendri*): drains damp heat, quells kidney fire, and detoxifies fire poisons.
- Anemarrhena (*zhi mu, Radix anemarrhenae asphodeloidis*): quells fire, nurtures yin, moistens dryness, and clears deficiency heat.

- Oyster shell (*mu li, Concha ostrea*): calms the spirit, benefits the yin, restrains rising yang, and restrains sweating.
- *Dang gui* (*tang kwei, Radix angelica sinensis*): tonifies the blood and invigorates and harmonizes the blood.

Notes Two Immortals is unusual in that it employs kidney yang strengthening herbs to treat a kidney yin deficiency. This is like treating fire with fire, instead of treating fire with water. Oddly enough, it works. The proportion of ingredients in the Dr. Shen's version of this formula is adjusted to further restrain rising heat and astringe sweating in order to better treat the hot flashes and sweats common to women in the West. The formula contains no estrogen or other hormones, and possibly achieves its effect by using yang tonics to help normalize hormone production.

Xanthium-Based Allergy Formulas

Dr. Shen's Sinus Pills; *Pe Min Kan Wan*, Chinese Patent Medicine; *Cang Er Zi Wan*, Plum Flower Brand

The common cocklebur fruit is called *cang er zi* in Chinese. Its botanical name is *Fructus xanthium*, and its use in subduing nasal allergies is well described in Chinese medical literature. The herb is absolutely safe when used in the above products, but can be mildly toxic when consumed raw.

Traditional Uses For nasal and sinus discomforts caused by allergic rhinitis or allergic sinusitis

Formula Functions in Chinese Medicine Terms The three formulas expel wind, relieve surface, drain dampness, alleviate pain, open the channels, release muscles, and circulate Qi and blood in the head.

Source The three formulas above are adapted from the formula Xanthium Powder and Magnolia Flower Powder, first published in *Formulas to Aid the Living* by Yan Hong He, 1253 AD.

Dosage Taken as a pill or powder, the dose is three to six grams per day (about one-ninth to one-fifth of an ounce). Taken as a boiled decoction, the dose is fifteen to thirty grams per day (about one-half to one ounce per day). Some versions of this formula contain the fruit of *Liquidambar styraciflua*, which is not recommended for pregnancy in larger amounts. In the context of this formula, however, the small dosage is regarded as safe.

Suggestions Xanthium-Based Allergy Formulas address the symptomatic aspect of disease, known as the Branch. To treat the deeper, causative aspect of the disease, known as the Root, see a qualified practitioner of Chinese Medicine. For year-round or persistent allergies made worse by stress, combine with equal amounts of *xiao yao wan* (Free and Easy Pills).

Ingredients and Functions The three formulas contain different variations of the following herbs:
- Cocklebur fruit (*cang er zi, Xanthium fructus*): opens the nasal passages, disperses wind, expels dampness, and relieves discharge.
- Magnolia bud (*xin ye hua, Magnolia flos*): expels wind, relieves surface, and opens nasal passages.
- Patchouli plant (*huo xiang, Agastach pogostemi*): transforms dampness, releases the exterior, harmonizes the center, and expels dampness.
- Kudzu root (*ge gen, Pueraria radix*): clears heat, releases muscles of upper body, and nourishes fluids.
- Chrysanthemum flower (*ju hua, Chrysanthemomi flos*): disperses wind, clears heat from the eyes, and pacifies the liver.
- Lovage root (*chuan xiong, Liguisticum wallichi szechuan*): invigorates the blood, circulates Qi, and alleviates pain.
- Liquidambar fruit (*lu lu tong, Liquidambar fructus*): promotes the flow of Qi and blood, unblocks the channels, opens the middle burner, and mollifies allergic sensitivity.
- Angelica root (*bai zhi, Angelica dahurica*): expels wind, releases surface, alleviates pain, reduces swelling, expels dampness, and alleviates discharge.

Notes These formulas contain no *ma huang* or synthesized ephedrine and will not cause drowsiness or agitation. They are for symptomatic relief only, to be used as needed. Tablets are most potent when taken on an empty stomach and given at least half an hour to digest alone before food or other supplements are taken. If the user experiences digestive difficulties, tablets should be taken with food

Formula Dynamics of Dr. Shen's Sinus Pills The chief herbs, *Xanthium fructus* (*cang er zi*), *Angelica dahurica* (*bai zhi*, and *Magnolia flos* (*xin yi hua*) unblock the sinuses and the nasal passages. These herbs are assisted by *Liquidamber fructus* (*lu lu tong*), which mollifies allergic sensitivity, while chrysanthemum (*ju hua*) and kudzu root (*ge gen*) pacify uprising heat and release the muscles of the head.

Adjunctive herb *Agastach pogostemi* (*huo xiang*) adjusts the dispersement of fluids, and Liguisticum wallichi szechuan (*chuan xiong*) is used to circulate Qi and blood and as a messenger to direct the formula to the head.

Good Sleep and Worry-Free Pill

Dr. Shen's Shui De An; United Pharmaceutical Factory, Guangzhou

Good Sleep and Worry-Free Pill is used to relieve insomnia or anxiety caused by disturbed *shen*, which in turn has been caused by deficiencies of heart blood or heart yin. This may sound esoteric; however, these conditions are very common and account for the majority of insomnia cases.

Traditional Use For disturbed *shen*: the word *shen* means "spirit," and "disturbed *shen*" indicates that the spirit is unsettled and is agitating the mind and nervous system. Good Sleep and Worry-Free Pill is used for a wide range of disturbed-shen conditions including insomnia, anxiety, dream-disturbed sleep, irritability, restlessness, or a rancorous disposition. Some practitioners also use it to treat attention deficit disorder. This formula contains no heavy metal mineral stabilizers, such as loadstone, oyster shell, or cinnabar, which are used in some other Chinese herbal sleep remedies. This makes Good Sleep

and Worry-Free Pill safe for long-term use and safe for use by pregnant or nursing women.

Source Twentieth century patent medicine.

Dosage In powders or pills, take three to six grams daily, plus an
extra three grams when awake at night. Use five times this quantity
for whole herb decoctions.

Course of Use One week or longer. Results are usually obtained
after three to seven days of regular use.

Suggestions This formula is not considered to cause drowsiness
or impair mental or physical functions; nevertheless, each person's
reaction should be assessed before performing potentially hazardous
activities such as driving or operating machinery.

Ingredients and Chinese Medicine Functions
- Sour date seed (*suan zao ren, Zizyphus semen*): nourishes the heart
  and calms the spirit.
- Chinese sage root (*dan shen, Salvia radix*): clears heat from the
  heart, invigorates the heart blood.
- Siberian milk wort (*zhi mu, Anemarrhena radix*): clears heat, quells
  fire, and tonifies the yin.
- Arbor vitae seed (*bai zhi ren, Biota semen*): nourishes the heart
  and calms the spirit.
- Atractylodes root (*bai zhu, Atractylodes radix*): tonifies the spleen
  and aids the assimilation of the formula.
- Schizandra fruit (*wu wei zi, Schisandra fructus*): astringes the essence and calms the spirit.
- Heart of poria (*fu ling, Poria cocos*): calms the spirit and aids
  the digestion and assimilation of the formula's yin tonics.
- Gardenia seed (*zhi zi, Gardenia semen*): clears heat from the
  heart and relieves irritability and restlessness.
- Bulrush (*deng xin cam, Medula junci*): drains heart heat and
  relieves insomnia.
- Ginseng root (*ren shen, Panax ginseng rx*): benefits the heart Qi,
  calms the spirit, and tonifies original Qi.

- Chinese licorice root (*gan cao, Glycyrrhiza radix*): aids in the assimilation of (harmonizes) other herbs.

Today there is much commentary that U.S. consumer purchases are making China rich. Though this might be true, these treasures of advanced herbal medicine may provide an inadvertent payback. Once these medicines are tried, recognized, and adopted by people in the Western world, they may outperform and replace many of the drugs now endangering individual health, while saving futile trips to the doctor. If health is wealth, these medical gems can bring richness.

6

Treatment of Ailments A to Z

This chapter explains how each of these common ailments is seen through the eyes of practitioners of Chinese medicine. Chinese medical practitioners view these ailments differently, seeing many modern diseases as amalgams of several underlying illnesses. For example, to the practitioner of traditional Chinese medicine, a simple head cold has at least two causes: one is a virus, and the other is a failed immune system.

The causes and treatment options according to Chinese medical practices are provided for each ailment. General comments are offered about how useful acupuncture may or may not be for a particular condition. Specific herbal treatment options are provided according to the Chinese medical diagnosis. In some instances, the ingredients of herbal formulas are listed so that you may prepare them yourself. However, since many prefer the convenience of ready-made herbal medicines, every attempt was made to list products that are widely available, and to list one or more manufacturer of each herbal medicine. Chinese patent medicines are freely available online. Virtually everything mentioned in this book is available from www.drshen.com. Dr. Shen's and Plum Flower products are also available in many retail stores. A list of the major American and Chinese manufacturers of herbal medicines is provided in the resources section of the appendices.

Some people are afraid to use Chinese herbs because they have been warned about impurities. These fears have almost no basis, and have been blown far out of proportion. Thousands of people die from Western over-the-counter medicines every year. Very few die from herbs of any kind.

This chapter recommends only herbal medicines that have been safely used for at least fifty years. It avoids unproven combinations of Chinese herbs with Western drugs, and those with herbs not normally used in Chinese medicines. For detailed information on the purity and cleanliness of Chinese herbs, see Appendix 3, "The Processing and Purity of Chinese Herbs."

Acne

Disease Condition Acne and many other inflammatory skin diseases are symptoms of internal heat and damp. Resolving these conditions requires finding the sources of excess heat and dampness. When the causes remain, a complete resolution is not possible. But herbs and acupuncture can clear heat and drain dampness, relieving the conditions.

Heat and Dampness Versions Heat, according Chinese medical philosophy, refers both to heat you can measure, like a fever, and heat you cannot measure, like a hot flash. Heat sets matters in motion and triggers activity. Heat shows as inflammation, hyperactivity, or over-stimulation. Heat can come from irritating chemicals, foreign organisms, or by the friction caused by the constrained flow of Qi (energy). Heat is also the by-product of our metabolism and our digestion. Hormonal activity causes and is stimulated by heat. An overly stimulating diet can cause excess heat, as can a hyperactive mind or lifestyle. Since friction, caused by the emotional constraint of Qi, causes heat, frustration and emotional friction are considered to cause heat.

Our skin presents the symptom of heat as rashes, pimples, infections, redness, and other skin inflammations. Sometimes heat is caused by blood deficiency. When the blood is insufficient in quantity or quality to dilute normal body wastes (toxins) transported in the blood, Toxic Heat in the Blood will result. This condition appears on the skin and will be diagnosed as acne or other inflammatory skin disease.

Dampness or excess damp indicates excessive water in the body's tissues. As all living things seek water, microorganisms, such as bacteria, fungus, and virus, thrive in excessively damp body environments. In the skin, excess damp can be seen as swellings, cysts, pimples, pus, and fluid discharges. Dampness is often caused by imperfect digestion that leads to water accumulation (spleen deficiency), or by a lack of body heat sufficient to cook off the water (spleen yang deficiency). Dampness can result when perspiration, urination, or breathing is insufficient to clear water from the body. Living in damp environments can also penetrate the body and cause internal dampness.

Herbal Treatments   Acne is best treated by experienced Chinese herbologists. For those who are unable to find a competent practitioner near them, the following formula and products are balanced to clear both heat and damp, and can be helpful in most cases. They are best taken for periods of three weeks or longer, and work best when heat from dietary sources is minimized.

Anti-Acne Products
- Margarite Anti-Acne pills: Plum Flower, Herbal Times, Fushan brands
- Complexion Pills: Dr. Shen brand
- Fang Feng Tong Sheng Wan: Plum Flower, Tanglong brand
- Acne Sweeping pill: Ching Tung Wing Medicine Co., Guangzhou
- Anti-Acne Formula: Combine nine grams each of the following herbs in four cups of water. Cover halfway and medium boil for thirty minutes, down to about two cups of medicine. Strain and

drink one cup in the morning and the other in the evening, prefer-ably on an empty stomach.

- Job's tears seeds: *yi yi ren*
- Poria mushroom: *fu ling*
- Phellodendrin bark: *huang bai*
- Tree peony root bark: *mu dan pi*
- Red peony root: *chi shao*
- Goldenthread root: *huang lian*
- Chinese licorice root: *gan cao*

Addictions: Alcohol, Nicotine, and Other Substances

Non-Herbal Treatments Acupuncture was used to treat opium ad-dictions in China before 1890 and nicotine addictions in the United States since about 1980, when its use as a stop-smoking aid became generally known. Substance abuse treatments usually involve auricular acupuncture, in which small fine needles are placed in the ear to help tranquilize the patient and help reduce cravings. Studies in prisons and other institutions have tested its effectiveness in curtailing the use of heroin and cocaine, with generally positive results. Type "acupuncture and substance abuse" into your favorite search engine for the latest in-formation on these studies.

Despite its success in institutional settings, I have had mixed results in my own practice using acupuncture to cure addictions. I have regular success with tobacco smokers, but almost none with other forms of ad-diction. Perhaps the difference is that treatment is enforced on a regular basis, often daily, in an institution such as a prison or halfway house, and participation is free and easy. Outside, it is rare to find addicts with the financial resources or motivation to get acupuncture three or more times a week; hence, sporadic, unconnected treatments become ineffective.

Herbal Treatments Treatment of addictions with Chinese herbal medicine is less well known but may offer promise. At the turn of the last century, a huge percentage of the Chinese population was addict-ed to opium. Chinese medicine played a key role in its irradiation, along with the wholesale execution of traffickers. One of the chief formulas given to addicts of that time was called Fog Tea of Tianmu Mountain, which is sold today under the brand name Westlake Stop Smoking Tea (*xi hu jie yan cha*), produced by the China National Pharmaceutical Factory. You can find it at any Chinese herb shop or online.

For those with alcohol addictions, *ge gen* and *ge hua* (kudzu root and kudzu flowers) have been used in East Asia to treat drunkenness and intoxication. Tests at Harvard Medical School concluded that the compounds in kudzu offer promise as effective agents for alcohol abuse.

Use as tea on a regular basis for three to five weeks for this purpose. Roots and flowers can both be used or combined. Flowers are steeped or quickly boiled. Roots should be boiled for thirty to forty minutes. Powdered concentrate can be stirred into liquid.

Other formulas and products said to calm the spirit may be helpful for those fighting any kind of addiction. Appropriate formulas include:

- Free and Easy Pill: many brands available (see Chapter 5, "Famous Herbal Medicines").
- All *bu nao* formulas including:
    Healthy Brain Pill: Dr. Shen's, Tsingtao brands
    Cerebral Tonic Pill: Xian Pharmaceutical, Plum Flower brands

Allergies

Disease Condition   Practitioners of Chinese medicine have understood for several millennia that allergies have numerous underlying causes that differ for each person, yet produce similar reactions in each. Modern doctors believe in a singular medical condition known as "allergy" every time hypersensitivity to various substances is exhibited. Their "cure" offers drugs that suppress the body's reaction to "allergens" or recommendations to simply avoid them. Few doctors look deeper to understand why such reactions exist.

Non-Herbal Treatments   Resolving allergies with acupuncture and herbs is entirely possible as Chinese medicine allows practitioners to diagnose and treat root imbalances on an individual basis. Root problems that commonly combine and bloom into allergies include

Liver Qi Stagnation, Excess Heat, Wei Qi Vacuity, and Spleen Qi Deficiency. These patterns are discussed elsewhere in this book under the specific diseases they can provoke. When these underlying roots are resolved or rebalanced by treatment, allergic reactions often lessen as a consequence.

Herbal Treatments Skilled herbal counsel is recommended. Lacking such counsel, diagnosis, or cure, allergy sufferers can still find safe and sure temporary relief using over-the-counter Chinese medicines. Note that all these remedies deal with airborne allergies rather than food allergies. The term "food allergies" is broadly used by many modern day practitioners of holistic medicine who mistake the symptom for the disease. A diagnosis of food allergies by your MD, chiropractor, or other health professional merely states the obvious. Digging deeper, airborne and food allergies have root causes that must be diagnosed and treated according to the constitution and circumstances of the individual patient.

Individual herbs that can also be combined into formulas (making them safer and more effective) to treat airborne allergies include:
- Xanthium: *cang er zi*
- Lquidambar: *lu lu tong*
- Angelica dahurica: *bai zhi*
- Asarum: *xi xin*
- Astragalus: *huang qi*

Over-the-counter herbal remedies for airborne allergies include:
- Magnolia Flower pills (*xin yi wan*): Herbal Times, other imported brands
- Sinus and Nose pills (*pe min kan wan*): Dr. Shen's
- Allergy pills (*min kan wan*): Dr. Shen's
- Xanthium Powder pills (*cang er zi wan*): Plum Flower brand
- Nasal Pain pills (*bi tong wan*): Herbal Times, Bio Essence brands
- Nasal Susceptibility pill (*pe min kan wan*): many versions available

Alzheimer's

Disease Condition Alzheimer's disease represents about 75 percent of all cases of senile dementia in the United States. The disorder is marked by development of amyloid plaques and degeneration of brain tissue. Alzheimer's usually occurs after the age of sixty. Symptoms of Alzheimer's disease and most forms of dementia, such as loss of memory and irritability, are understood by Chinese medicine to be associated with the kidneys or the heart. Modern medical treatment involves use of hydergine, dexedrine, and antidepressant drugs. In Europe, there is widespread use of Ginkgo biloba leaf for this condition.

Notes In China, one of the most promising modern day herbal treatments for Alzheimer's disease involves Huperzine A, an alkaloid extracted from the herb *Huperzia serotta*, which inhibits the breakdown of the neurotransmitter acetylcholine, increasing neurotransmission in the body. Though one can't get enough Huperzine A by simply consuming the whole herb, certain traditional Chinese herbs and herbal formulas may also significantly increase levels of acetylcholine. Coptis (*huang lian*) is one such herb.

Seeing a practitioner skilled in the use of Chinese herbs is important.

For those unable to find a practitioner near them, the herbs *zizyphus, biota, polygala*, and *acorus* are traditionally used to treat heart disorders involving memory. Kidney tonics such as *jin gui shen qi wan* or *mai wei di huang wan* (see Chapter 5, "Famous Herbal Medicines") should be added.

Herbal Treatments

- Healthy Brain pills: *bu nao wan*
- Good Sleep and Worry Free pills: *shui di an*
- Emperor's Tea pills: *tian huang bu xin wan*

Arthritis, Bursitis, Tendonitis, and Joint Pain

Joint pains are mostly diagnosed as arthritis, bursitis, or tendonitis by modern physicians. Tendonitis is joint pain without signs of calcification, while arthritis is characterized by calcification or joint disfigurement. Joint pain originating in the bursa, the protective envelope that surrounds a joint, is called bursitis.

This differentiation is largely irrelevant to the acupuncturist or acupressure massage therapist, who sees that whether the pain emanates from the tendon, the bursa, or the muscle, his or her role is simply to restore normal flow, and the selection of points will be similar no matter what body tissues are involved. However, the acupuncturist or herbologist will also focus on the conditions that have resulted in this problem. A diagnosis of arthritis leads us to suspect the usual patterns: Bi Syndrome, Liver Not Smoothing the Qi, Deficiency of Liver Yin, and Third-Stage Injuries. They all look like arthritis, bursitis, or tendonitis to your doctor. These conditions, which can exist in combination, obstruct flow in the joints, potentially causing inflammation, calcification, and joint pain.

Treating arthritis, tendonitis, or bursitis effectively with Chinese herbs requires diagnosing which of the above conditions is the probable cause of the "arthritis," then choosing the correct course of treatment. Diagnosis is made according to the Four Examinations (see Chapter 2, "A Patient's Guide to Acupuncture and Herbs"). Professional help is highly recommended in making this diagnosis for herbal treatment. Acupuncture can be very effective for all of the following conditions.

Cause #1 of Arthritis/Tendonitis/Bursitis: Bi-Syndrome

Bi Syndrome indicates that our defensive energy (wei qi) has become weak, allowing weather-related conditions to penetrate our bodies, thus obstructing flow and causing pain or stiffness. When arthritis is sensitive to the weather, the patient is likely have Bi Syndrome. Four kinds are recognized depending on what types of weather make symptoms worse: hot bi, cold bi, damp bi, and windy bi. Treatment plans typically involve expelling the evil Qi (pathogenic influence), relieving pain, and boosting the wei Qi.

Hot Bi Syndrome is usually diagnosed as rheumatoid arthritis or gouty arthritis, but may also be identified as tendonitis or bursitis. Joints can look red or feel hot. Putting heat on such an inflamed joint makes it feel worse. Treatment protocols for this condition include Moving Blood, Clearing Heat, and Restoring the Yin Fluids of the Joints. Often this condition evolves through periods of heat and cold and must be treated differently as it progresses.

Both cold bi and damp bi are usually diagnosed as osteoarthritis. Joints may be stiff, painful, or disfigured. They feel better when heat is applied. Moxibustion is often used (see Chapter 3, "Understanding Theories of Chinese Medicine"). Cold bi gets worse in cold weather. Damp bi gets worse during periods of damp weather and fog. When cold bi or damp bi sufferers go to a warm, dry climate, they often feel much better.

Windy bi acts like the wind. Pain migrates around the body. Like the wind, it can spring up and subside quickly. Last week it was shoulder pain, this week the knees hurt. Symptoms of windy bi may appear the same as cause #2: the liver is not smoothing the Qi.

Cause #2 of Arthritis/Tendonitis/Bursitis: Liver Not Smoothing the Qi   A function of the liver, according to Chinese theory, is to insure the smoothness of flow. When damage or stress to this organ occurs, its ability to insure smooth flow may be impaired. Since the liver also governs the joints and tendons, liver patterns can cause pain in the joints and tendons. The Chinese diagnosis in these cases is Liver Not Smoothing the Qi.

Cause #3 of Arthritis/Tendonitis/Bursitis: Liver Yin Deficiency
Yin deficiencies are usually accompanied by a shortage of fluids. Since the liver governs the joints and tendons, liver yin deficiencies result in a reduction of the synovial fluids that lubricate the joints and tendons. The loss of lubrication and subsequent increased friction can cause joint pain and be diagnosed as arthritis, bursitis, or tendonitis.

Cause #4 of Arthritis/Tendonitis/Bursitis: Third-Stage Injury
Old injuries that have not healed properly also restrict the flow-through of Qi and blood. Restricted flow, over time, causes the accumulations and deposits that invite a diagnosis of arthritis. These weak flows also result in poor nourishment and subsequent weakening of the injured area.

Herbal Treatments   The following table shows a few of the medicines used to treat joint pain. These formulas are safe and widely available in pill form. However, many contain herbs that should be avoided by pregnant women. Herbs are almost always used in formulas. Most substances used to counter Bi Syndrome (arthritis) belong to the category Herbs to Expel Wind and Damp. Single herbs are:

- White patterned snake (*bai hua she, Agkistrodon*)
- Duhuo root (*du huo, Angelicae pubescens radix*)
- Sea paulownia bark (*hai tong pi, Erythrinae cortex*)
- Papaya (*mu gua, Chaenomelis fructus*)
- Silkworm excrement (*can sha, Bombycis faeces*)
- Gentian root (*Qin jiao, Gentianae macrophyllae*)
- Chinese clematis root (*wei ling xian, Clematidis radix*)
- White or red peony root (*bai shao* or *chi shao, Peonea alba* or *rubra*)

Non-Herbal Treatments of Chinese Medicine   Acupuncture, moxibustion, and acupressure massage are effective in treating arthritis, bursitis, and tendonitis. These modalities aggressively promote the movement of Qi and blood to relieve pain and promote normalcy. Moxibustion (heat treatment) is extremely beneficial in treating cold conditions such as cold bi, damp bi, and third-stage injuries. Moxibustion is inappropriate in hot conditions, such as when a joint appears red or feels warm to the touch, or in cases of rheumatoid arthritis.

	#1 Bi Syndrome	#2 Liver Not Smoothing the Qi
Internal Medicines	Hot Bi: Feng Shih Shiao Tung Wan Cold Bi: Zhen Wu Wan (True Warrior Pills) Damp Bi: Xuan Bi Wan (Clear Channels Pill) Windy Bi: Feng Shi Ding Pill	Xiao Yao San Linking Decoction plus *niu xi* and *yi yi ren*
Topical Medicines	Zheng Gu Shui Hua Tuo Rheumatism Plaster	Topicals not often helpful

Asthma

Disease Condition   Modern MDs have a single diagnosis—asthma—for what practitioners of traditional Chinese medicine diagnose as four different conditions:

- Spleen Deficiency, which creates dampness in the lung
- Liver Heat, which scorches the lung

- Lung Qi Deficiency, which results in lung weakness
- Kidney Qi Deficiency, which leave the lungs unable to grasp the Qi

Effective treatment with herbs depends on diagnosing which condition is the root cause of the asthma. This can be a challenge, as two or more causes may be involved, and because conditions evolve over time. This can mean different prescriptions for the same person at different times. When you can't find a good Chinese herbologist in your area, here are some recommendations that are generally available in pill form.

Spleen Deficiency Asthma is often characterized by excess mucous. The condition is called spleen deficiency, but has nothing to do with your physical spleen. Rather, it is caused by a constitutional or digestive deficiency, which, among other things, causes the body to hold on to water. The excess water can become mucous and often affects the lungs. This "dampness" can also affect the nose and sinuses, which are considered part of the lung and are a favorite collection site for dampness. A simple and highly effective herbal formula for this condition when it produces a watery sputum affecting the lungs is *er chen wan*.

#3 Deficiency of Liver or Kidney Yin	#4 Old Injury
Linking Decoction Liu Wei Di Huang Qi Ju Di Huang Golden Book Pill	China Tung Shui Pills Chin Koo Tieh Shang Pills Qi Ye Lian Pills
Topicals not often helpful	Tieh Ta Yao Gin Zheng Gu Shui Plaster for bruise

Heat Scorching the Lungs Asthma, which presents with thick phlegm, green phlegm, no phlegm, or no cough, may be caused by heat in the body that has reached the lungs. Heat can come from outside your body. Pollution, alcohol, microorganisms, allergens, drugs, and food are potential sources of exterior heat. Heat can also come from within. Emotional stress or fluid deficiencies, such as yin or blood deficiencies, are potential sources of heat from within, called interior heat.

Herbal Treatments The patent medicine *ching fei yi huo* effectively addresses many of these conditions, often within a day, when they are in an acute phase. However, this Chinese medicine is not recommended for long-term use or for pregnant women or nursing mothers.

Any type of asthma sufferer can take a Chinese herbal tablet called *ma hsing chih ke pian*, taken together with an early stage cold tablet such as *gan mao ling* or *yin chiao*.

Lung weakness, another cause of asthma, may exist alone or accompany other root causes. This deficiency can stem from childhood, or appear later after the lung has been damaged by cold, flu, or other assault. Lung weakness comes with or without a cough. It is sometimes accompanied by fatigue, shortness of breath, weak voice, shallow breathing, heart palpitations, catching colds easily, and other signs of general debility. This condition requires long-term treatment. Dry lung pill and Ping Chuan pills are both recommended.

Kidney-deficient asthma sometimes comes with lower back pain. Weakness, debility, or fatigue can also be present. This kind of asthma indicates that the lungs are starved of energy normally obtained from the kidney, energy needed to extract Qi from the air. Because the kidneys are weak, the lungs function poorly. This asthma will worsen when the sufferer gets tired or drained of Qi. The Chinese patent formula *ge ji da bu wan* can be used together with *ping chuan wan* to improve this condition.

ADD, ADHD, and Compulsive Behavior

Disease Condition In the literature of Traditional Chinese Medicine, prominent symptoms of Attention Deficit Disorder (ADD) are associated with a syndrome known as Deficiency of Heart Blood or Deficiency of Heart Yin. Restlessness, poor concentration, hyperactivity, anxiety, compulsive behavior, disturbed sleep, and other changes in consciousness are associated with this condition.

Non-Herbal Treatments In many cases, acupuncture can be helpful as it can be extremely relaxing, helping to calm and sedate a mind made restless due to these heart deficiencies. Needles will likely be placed on the scalp, chest, and the insides of the forearm. Note that these are fluid deficiencies, not energetic ones, and so do not affect the function (yang) of the heart. They therefore do not portend serious heart disease of any kind.

Herbal Treatments Herbal treatment will probably include herbs from one or more of the following categories:
- Herbs that tonify heart blood
- Herbs that tonify heart yin
- Herbs that tonify the spleen
- Herbs that open the orifices
- Herbs that drain heart fire

Herbal Medicines for Memory and Concentration (ADD/ADHD) The following packaged medicines have been chosen because they contain no heavy mineral stabilizers and may be easily found online or in Chinatowns throughout North America and Europe.
- Healthy brain pills: Dr. Shen's
- Cerebral tonic pills: Chinese patent medicine
- *Tian huan bu xin tang:* Chinese patent medicine
- *Gui pi wan*: Chinese patent medicine
- Acorus tablets: Seven Forests

Single Herbs for Memory and Concentration (ADD/ADHD)
- Longan fruit (*long yan rou*)
- Chinese dates (*da zao*)
- Chinese date seed (*suan zao ren*)
- Sweetflag (s*hi chang pu*)

Back Pain

Disease Condition Where Western doctors see a solid nerve, practitioners of Chinese medicine visualize the flow of energy (Qi) as flow in a channel. Many of these channels pass through your back, activating your muscles and nourishing your spine. To the practitioner of Chinese medicine, pain means that flow is impaired. The obstruction may be visible or invisible. Chiropractors can sometimes relieve back pain by adjusting the vertebra, freeing the flow of Qi, but adjustments may not always correct the cause of this aberrant Qi.

Acupuncturists and Chinese herbologists often heal back pain when others fail because practitioners of Traditional Chinese Medicine work to understand what influences the Qi. They know that body structures will ultimately conform to the Qi.

Several Causes of Back Pain

Channel Pain: Stuck Qi, Flow No Go There are at least ten separate flows of energy traversing the back. Much back pain is a sign of obstruction or constraint of Qi in the channels. Old or new injuries, emotional constraint, anatomical obstructions, and other events can constrain the Qi in the channels.

Upper Back Pain: Excess Qi, Congested Heat Heat rises, and upper back pain is commonly caused by interior heat that rises in the channels and lodges in the neck, shoulders, and head, causing tension in the muscles. A commonly used herbal formula for this condition is Pueraria Combination (ge gen tang). A tablet version is Pueraria 10 tablets.

Lower Back Pain: Weak Qi, Low Batteries The lower back is the domain of the kidney. As the kidneys store much of our Qi, we experience this stored energy in our lower back. Stored Qi in the lower back keeps our back strong, and holds the spine erect. Depletion of this energy weakens the lower back, making injuries more likely to occur. Stress, injury, illness, overwork, excessive sex, drugs, and overstimulation of the brain drain the kidney Qi and weaken the lower back. The most often used formula for any kind of lower back or lower body pain is *du huo ji shen wan*. This formula is excellent for helping circulation in the lower body, but its action as a kidney strengthener is mild. Kidney deficiencies come in different forms, and are not always easy for professionals to diagnose. Rather than ponder yin from yang, it's best to choose a kidney strengthener (tonic) that is comprehensive and builds several qualities of energy.

Herbal Treatments *Gui fu di huang wan* is also known as *jin gui di huang wan*, Golden Book pills, or Sexoton pills. Having so many names testifies to its ancient and widespread use. It is easily available anywhere Chinese herbs are sold (see Chapter 5, "Famous Herbal Medicines").

If you are able to distinguish yin from yang and you know that your deficiency is clearly a kidney yang deficiency, with accompanying signs of coldness, remedies such as You Gui Wan (returning the right side), and Chuang Chuang Yao Tonic pills are useful as well.

When kidney yin deficiency is diagnosed with accompanying signs of warmth or heat, it can be treated with Liu Wei Di Huang, Zhi Bai Di Huang, or Da Bu Yin wan. They also are described in Chapter 5 ,"Famous Herbal Medicines." Another very useful formula, also widely available, is Zuo Gui Wan (returning the left side pills). Several variations of this formula are on the market. Though classified as yin tonics, these formulas strengthen both the yin and yang Qi.

Bleeding Disorders

Disease Condition In Chinese medicine, blood disorders fall into three main categories: bleeding, stagnant blood, and deficient blood.

Herbal Treatments Logically, there are three categories of herbs to treat these three conditions: herbs that stop bleeding, herbs that move or vitalize the blood, and herbs that tonify the blood.

When treating bleeding problems with herbs, there are additional factors to consider, such as the location and cause of the bleeding, and the constitution of the patient. It must be kept in mind that most herbs used internally to stop bleeding can have a stagnating effect when used long-term. If the bleeding is external due to traumatic injury, *san qi* (pseudoginseng root, Radix notoginseng) is recommended. It is used both internally and topically to stem bleeding caused by trauma. It is used alone or found in various combinations. Perhaps the most effective is the popular formula Yunnan Baiyao, available as powder, capsules, and skin patches wherever Chinese herbs are sold.

Treating bleeding disorders not caused by trauma is much more complicated. Getting professional help is advised. However, obtaining a modern medical diagnosis does not tell the whole story. A bleeding disorder identified by Western medicine might have different causes in different people. Retinal bleeding can be caused by excess in some and deficiency in others. Abnormal menstrual bleeding can have a dozen different causes. A persistent bloody nose can indicate a serious disorder, or mean little. Practitioners of Chinese medicine seek the cause of the bleeding with the treatment goal of harmonizing the body to stop the symptoms. Bleeding disorders caused by weakness must be distinguished from those caused by excess, and the particular nature of these imbalances must also be deciphered, hot from cold.

For example, cold-induced bleeding, often due to a spleen, yang, or blood deficiency, is treated with warming herbs like mugwort (*ai ye*). On the other hand, bleeding caused by heat (Reckless Marauding of Blood) is treated with cold herbs like *ce bai ye, huai hua mi*, and *da ji*.

When blood heat is combined with or caused by yin deficiency, the above individual herbs can be combined with *e jiao, han lian cao*, or *sheng di huang*. When spleen deficiency is the cause, herbs to tonify the spleen, such as Four Gentlemen tonic (see Chapter 5, "Famous Herbal Medicines"), are added to the formula. Other herbs used to stop bleeding include: human hair (*xue yu tan*), lotus receptacle (*lian fang*) and pollen (*pu huang*). The most popular herb, used for both traumatic and deficiency-caused bleeding disorders, is pseudoginseng root (*san Qi* or *tian Qi*).

Products Used to Stop Bleeding

Pseudoginseng (san qi, tian chi, tinchi) Stops bleeding without promoting clotting, reduces swelling, and alleviates pain. Taoist monks use it as a life-extender and general tonic. North Vietnamese soldiers used it during the Vietnam War. Do not use during pregnancy.

Yunnan Paiyao (also spelled Yunnan Baiyao) Stops bleeding, and promotes the healing of wounds. Also helps excessive menstrual bleeding. Good for pre- and post-surgery. Keep on hand for emergencies. Use one to two caps three times a day or as needed. Use red pellet only for severe emergency bleeding. Do not use during pregnancy.

Cancer

Disease Condition Cancer is well documented in Chinese medical literature. Drawings of tumors have been found on turtle shells and "oracle bones" dating from the eleventh century BC. Medical texts dating from 200 BC have detailed descriptions of tumors and their causes. Yet there is no word for cancer in this literature. Practitioners of Chinese medicine have always regarded cancer as several different diseases rather than as a single ailment. Modern physicians are starting to come to the same conclusion.

Notes It is hard to find advice on using Chinese herbs to treat cancer. Cancer therapies are not generally taught to undergraduates at most schools of Chinese medicine in the United States or Europe. Therefore, this section is meant both for the education of patients without access to professional help and as an introduction for acupuncturists and other holistic practitioners.

As mentioned above, Chinese medical treatment of cancer is based on the principle of *fu zheng gu ben*. *Fu zheng* means strengthening what is correct. *Gu ben* means regeneration and repair.

Every disease, according to Chinese medical philosophy, including cancer, must have at least two causes. One group of causes is the pathogenic factors. These are the forces that cause disharmony, the assault that disrupts the status quo. In the case of cancer, these causes often take the form of irritants. They may originate from outside or inside the body. These toxic irritants place stress upon the cells.

A second group of causes is the resistance factors. Various imbalances can weaken the body's defenses. Any treatment for cancer would be incomplete without taking this into account. Disregarding the body's defense system is like using yang and ignoring yin. The results would be less than perfect.

In many cancers, there is a third cause: the flow factor. Chinese medicine is about flow. When flow of Qi and blood is normal, body functions and structures tend to be normal or to eventually normalize. These cleansing flows can be seen as part of the body's defense system as they function to circulate toxic impurities (heat) throughout our bodies and thus reduce their potential for stressing any particular part of the body. When these normal flows are impaired, accumulations can result, including accumulations of cancer-provoking toxic heat.

Treating cancer with Chinese herbs, using the principle of *fu zheng gu ben*, means that the formula must correct the imbalance by rebalancing yin and yang, thus strengthening what is correct. The formula must also repair the damage and help regenerate normalcy in cell structure and function.

The aim of treatment is focused on harmonizing body function within the patient rather than attacking cancerous cells. Such attacks are best left to Western medicine, which continues to develop an arsenal of formidable weapons to kill cancer cells.

Herbal Treatments Since balancing and harmonizing must be a part of every formula, and each person reaches harmony in a different way, each formula should be unique. There are, however, various components that appear very often in any anticancer herbal formula.

Herbs to Reduce or Break Stagnation Good health depends on normal flows that are affected by physical, mental, and environmental influences. Cancer can occur when poor flow causes prolonged exposure to toxicity. The resulting accumulation (tumor) can be attacked with strong blood-breaking and anti-cancer herbs. Herbs will differ according to the type and location of the cancer. Commonly used substances include bitter orange (*zhi shi, Fructus aurantium*), turmeric (*yu jin, Tuber curcuma*), and other blood vitalizing herbs. Because many patients receive toxic chemotherapy, and toxicity may be a disease factor, anti-toxic herbs such as *bai hua she she cao* (*Herba oldenlandia*) or *yu xing cao* (*Herba houttuynia*) are often added.

Herbs to Strengthen and Balance the Body In the West, we are beginning to recognize our immune system and what its role might be in the cause and cure of many diseases, including cancer. Chinese medicine has recognized the immune concept for several thousand years. In that time, many ways have been devised to enhance the protective Qi (*wei Qi*), which must be heightened to subdue the cancering process. Commonly used herbs are reishi mushroom (*ling zhi, Ganoderma*) and milk vetch root (*huang Qi, Radix astragali*).

Herbs to Eliminate the Root Causes This class of herb is effective in eliminating the cause and preventing recurrence. Cancer is caused when stagnation and toxicity combine and overwhelm the body's normal Qi. This rarely happens suddenly, and is most often the result of extended conditions in the life of the sufferer. Looking at a person's life can sometimes reveal answers to these questions. Are stagnations caused by physical or emotional factors? Have toxins been introduced from the outside—or from the internal chemical factory? Are the normal Qi and the defensive Qi strong? When these questions can be answered, the underlying patterns must be changed. When herbs are used, they must reflect the unique pattern of an individual's root disharmonies and cannot be prescribed for all people with cancer.

Anti-Cancer Formulas
- Breast cancer: *oldenlandia* (sixty grams), *Taraxacum* (sixty grams), *scutellaria* (sixty grams), *aurantium* (sixty grams), *curcuma* (sixty grams)
- Stomach cancer: combine *oldenlandia* (ninety grams) and *imperata* (sixty grams), or use *scutellaria* (thirty grams) and *Imperata* (thirty grams)
- Esophageal cancer: *oldenlandia* (sixty grams), *Scutellaria* (sixty grams), *imperata* (sixty grams), *cotton root* (sixty grams)
- Colon cancer: *oldenlandia* (sixty grams), *scutellaria* (fifteen grams), *solanum* (sixty grams), *sanguisorba* (thirty grams), *viola* (fifteen grams)
- Ovarian cancer: *oldenlandia* (thirty grams), *scutellaria* (fifty grams), *solanum* (fifty grams), turtle shell (thirty grams)
- Lung cancer: *scutellaria* (120 grams), *taraxacum* (thirty grams),

ophiopogonis (thirty grams), *oldenlandia* (sixty grams)
- Liver cancer: *oldenlandia* (sixty grams), *scutellaria* (sixty grams), *phragmites* (thirty grams), *peonae alba* (sixty grams)

Chinese Herbs Commonly Used in Treatment of Cancer

Vitalize Blood and/or Qi Herbs	Anti-Cancer Herbs	Strengthening Herbs	Miscellaneous Herbs
chih ko aurantium	*reishi* various mushrooms	*huang qi* Astragalu	*yi yi ren* coix
e zhu curcuma zedoaria	*lu feng fang* hornet's nest	*xi yang shen* American ginseng	*lugen* phragmites
tao ren persicae semen	*long kui* solanum	*shu di huang* Chinese foxglove root	*bai mao gen* imperata
hong hua Carthami tinctori	*ban zhi lian* Scutellaria	*gan cao* Chinese licorice root	*mu li* oyster shell, other shells
san leng sparganii rhizoma	*dong ling cao* rabdosime rubescentis	*dang gui* angelica sinensis	*pu gong yin* taraxacum
wu ling shi trogopterori pteromi	*bai hua she she cao* oldenlandia	*bie jia* turtle shell	*ji xue tengmillettia*

Dosages and the administration of these herbs is best charted by an experienced practitioner. Seek professional help for these conditions, and avoid self medication.

Herbs Used to Treat the Side Effects of Chemotherapy and Radiation

The side effects of chemotherapy and radiation are not the same for everyone. Different chemicals, people, and diseases mean that each case must be assessed separately. Practitioners offer the following suggestions for those with no access to professional help:

- Nausea: Curing Pills, or Dr. Shen's Stomach Curing pills
- Lowered Immunity: Jade Shield pills, Astragalus extract
- Dryness: Mai Wei Di Huang
- Radiation Burn: Jing Wan Hong ointment

- Low Libido: Man's Treasure for men, Two Immortals for women
- Flu-like symptoms (tidal fever, scratchy throat): Zhi Bai Di Huang

High Cholesterol

The following anti-cholesterol remedies are not taken from historical Chinese medicine. You would not find a word about cholesterol in any of the classics, as this substance was only discovered in modern times. The herbs are old and well established as safe. Their use in lowering cholesterol, however, is recent. There is a curious similarity between the ancient and the modern idea that obstructions in flow are the cause of heart attacks and strokes.

Disease Condition The modern understanding is that fatty blood (flowing with too much high cholesterol) can cause obstructions in the form of plaques that grow in the blood vessels, narrowing the channel and resulting in diminished blood flow to the heart and brain. This, coupled with blood clots that form in the vessels, can cause most cerebrovascular problems. Chinese doctors understood these patterns in a similar way. They knew that a thickened substance was obstructing the vessels, leading to a loss of consciousness. They called it Phlegm in the Channels Obstructing the Orifices. The signs of this condition are exactly those of stroke: loss of consciousness, paralysis, and loss of speech, among others (see Chapter 7, "Herbs and Their Categories").

Herbal Treatments The following Chinese herbs have been shown to reduce cholesterol in human beings. They are available wherever Chinese herbs are sold.

Hawthorn berry: shan za, Fructus crataegi This herb is sometimes called "haw" and is available in any Chinese food market. It is traditionally used as a digestive aid (see Chapter 5, "Famous Herbal Medicines").

Hawthorn fat reducing pills, Chinese patent medicine These are extracted from hawthorn berries with the sugar content removed.

In one clinical trial, cholesterol was reduced in 84.5 percent of the participants, triglyceride reduction was 77.39 percent, and hypertension due to hyperlipemia was reduced an astounding 97.2 percent. The herb has no side effects and can be administrated over long periods. The usual oral dose is one to two tablets three times a day, or two to three tablets twice a day. Minimum course of use is usually one month.

Jiao gu lan (jiao gu lian, jiaogulan) pills *Jiao gu lan* is an anti-aging, longevity tonic herb that strengthens the immune system. Chemically similar to ginseng, it reinforces overall health and has a strong anti-fatigue effect. It is used for a variety of health complaints including cholesterol reduction. It contains eighty-two saponins, some of which are directly related to the ginsenosides found in ginseng root. Minimum course of use is usually one month.

Cold and Flu

Non-Herbal Treatments Many of my patients benefit instantaneously from acupuncture when they have a cold. A few well-placed needles behind the neck on the gallbladder meridian at GB 20 (wind gate point) seems to quickly deflate the pressure in the head. A couple of ultra fine needles at the side of the nose (*bi tong* point) coupled with one in the hand on the liver meridian at LI 20 (*he gu* point) frees the stuck nasal Qi and drains it, along with the headache. On the other hand, many more people rely on Chinese herbs to prevent and treat cold or flu infections. Herbs are less expensive and probably more reliable than acupuncture for these conditions.

Notes Classical treatment of cold and flu with herbs is a difficult, highly technical procedure that requires the practitioner to diagnose the nature of the evil pathogen as well as the depth of its penetration. However, most cold and flu sufferers do not distinguish between a Wind Cold Evil and a Wind Heat Evil. Many of the Chinese herbal remedies traditionally used for Wind Heat conditions (flu or respiratory infection with high fever) will work most of the time for any cold or flu. Although some of these remedies are considered to work better at one stage of the disease or another, it varies from person to person.

Medicines in this category are generally meant for short-term use and are not intended for use over extended periods of time. Long-term use could damage the spleen, leading to digestive imbalances.

Herbal Treatments   There are hundreds of Chinese herbal products for cold and flu symptoms. Recent popular innovations mix Chinese herbs with popular herbs like goldenseal, echinacea, or elderberry; others contain mixtures of herbs and drugs. Since many of these newer mixtures have not yet withstood the test of time, I can recommend only the following remedies, which have proven to be remarkably effective. They are subcategorized as Stopping a Cold Early, Relieving a Cold, and Preventing a Cold (Bolstering Immunity).

Stopping a Cold Early

Yin Chiao   *Yin qiao*, Honeysuckle, Forsythia Clean Toxin pill
They say "bad news travels fast," so good news must travel slowly. In 1798, Dr. Wu Ju Tong first published the cold remedy *yin chiao*. He knew it worked because it had already been used for generations to ward off these hated infections.

Yin chiao may be as close as any product has come to curing the common cold. This remedy is 100 percent herbal, 100 percent safe, and though considered to be a remedy for Wind Heat conditions, it is proven to stop all kinds of colds and respiratory infections. It is a shame that it has taken Western cultures so long to discover it. You can find many brands of *yin chiao* wherever herbal medicines are sold. Dr. Shen's version is called ColdStop. You can ask for it at markets and pharmacies that don't ordinarily carry Chinese or herbal medicines.

Begin treatment at the first sign, or during the first two days, of cold or flu, or when you have been exposed or are likely to be exposed to cold or flu. Specific tips:
- Take promptly.
- Keep a dozen tablets in your car, purse, or pocket during cold and flu season.
- Begin taking tablets a half hour before entering airports, airplanes, movie theaters, or other crowded or confined spaces.

- For more information on this cold remedy, see Chapter 5, "Famous Herbal Medicines."

Gan Mao Ling Functions According to Chinese Medicine: clears heat, cleans toxins, dispels wind, relieves cough

How To Use Use alone or combined with *yin qiao* at the onset of cold or flu. Use *gan mao ling* alone or combined with *zong gan ling* for stronger relief of cold or flu symptoms. Use when cough or sinus congestion is present at the onset of a cold or flu.

Dosage Adults: When taken alone or together with *yin chiao* or *zong gan ling*, take two to four tablets every three to four hours.
Children: Crush one tablet for every twenty-five pounds of body weight. Mix with food or syrup.

Ingredients and Functions

- Lex root (*gang mei gen*): clears heat and resolves toxins
- Evodia leaf (*san cha ku*): clears heat and resolves toxins
- Chrysanthemum flower (*ju hua*): disperses wind heat, clears liver heat, and cools lung heat
- Vitex herb (*huang jing cao*): disperses wind heat, cools lung heat
- Isatis root (*ban lan gen*): clears heat, cleans toxins
- Lonicera flower (*jin yin hua*): clears heat, cleans toxins, and relieves the surface

Caution Because of the short history of use of some of its ingredients (less than 100 years), *gan mao ling* is not recommended for use during pregnancy.

Notes *Gan mao ling* can be used as a cold preventative alone or in combination with *yin chiao* at the *yangming* (early) stage of a cold or flu. It is also used alone or in combination with zong gan ling for added relief of symptoms in later stages. This formula may be most helpful for a cold or flu accompanied by a cough or sinus infection. However, do not use or prescribe this product for a dry cough that follows a respiratory infection, as a dry cough is usually caused by Lung Dryness. Use Dry Cough pills or Li Fei pills for these post-infection coughs. *Gan mao ling* is not an immune booster. Do not use it for extended periods (more than two weeks). For long-term immune enhancement use Jade Shield pills or Jade Windscreen powder.

Relieving a Cold

Zong Gan Ling Sometimes spelled *zhong gan ling*, this powerful formula is used for symptomatic relief of severe or advanced head cold or flu with symptoms such as headache, sore throat, nasal congestion, and body aches, fevers, and chills. The formula clears heat, drains dampness, eliminates cold, releases muscles, and relieves pain.

The exact source of this formula is anonymous. *Zhong gan ling*, previously manufactured by the Meizhou Pharmaceutical Manufactory in Guangdong, China, has since been banned because it contained an illegal pharmaceutical. You can still obtain the Dr. Shen's, Plum Flower, and Herbal Times versions, none of which contain the illegal drug, and all of which are effective and safe.

Dosage Adults: take one to three grams, three or four times a day; do not exceed twelve grams a day. Children: crush tablets and mix with food. Use one-half gram for every thirty pounds of body weight, three to four times a day.

Caution Use only when necessary, which is usually only for a few days. There is a prudent maximum of two weeks. Cold or flu symptoms lasting longer than two weeks require professional attention. Strong heat-clearing herbs such as these are not recommended as a daily supplement.

Ingredients and Functions
* Kudzu root (*ge gen, Radix puerariae*): clears heat, releases the muscles, and nourishes fluids.
* Hairy holly root (*mao tung ching, Radix illicis pubescentis*): clears toxic heat, and invigorates blood.
* Vervain (herb of the cross, *ma pien tsao, Herba verbenae*): clears heat and disperses blood.
* Woad root (indigo, *ban lan gen, Radix isatidis*): quells heat, detoxifies fire poison, and benefits the throat.
* Wormwood plant (*Qing hao, Herba artemisae*): clears heat, cools

blood, clears deficiency fever, and clears summer heat.

- Gypsum (*shi gao, Gypsum fibrosum*): quells fire, clears heat, and clears stomach fire rising to the head.
- Notopterygi (*Qiang huo, Radix* and *Rhizome notopterygium incisium*): releases the exterior, disperses cold and dampness, alleviates pain, and directs herbs upward.

Preventing a Cold (Bolstering Immunity)

Jade Shield or Jade Windscreen This formula is used to build defensive energy (*wei Qi*) and consolidate the surface (protect against cold, flu, and other illness-causing invasions).

Source Jade Windscreen Powder, *Teachings of Zhu Dan Xi*, 1481 AD

Functions According to Chinese Medicine: Augments the Qi, stabilizes the exterior, stops sweating. This formula is used for weak defensive energy (*wei qi*) leading to recurrent colds, low immunity, spontaneous sweating, sensitivity to wind, and other signs of lowered immunity. It can sometimes be useful for allergies or chronic rhinitis with clear mucous.

The Plum Flower and Herbal Times brands, as well as most other versions of this formula, contain *huang qi* (*Astragalus*), *bai zhu* (*Atractylodes*), and *fang feng* (*ledebouriella*). The Dr. Shen's Jade Shield version adds *nu zhen zi* (privet fruit)) and *gui zhi* (cinnamon twig) to expand the immune-enhancing property of the *Astragalus* while reducing the drying effects of the *Atractylodes* and the *ledebouriella*. These changes make the formula more suitable for long-term use for those with dry or yin-deficient constitutions.

Ingredients and Functions
- Milk vetch root (*huang qi, radix Astragalus membricanaceus*): sweet taste, warming temperature, benefits the Qi, lifts the yang, strengthens the spleen/pancreas, and tonifies the *wei Qi* (defensive energy).
- Privet fruit (*nu zhen zi, Ligustri lucidi fructus*): bitter and sweet taste, neutral temperature, nourishes and tonifies the liver and kidney yin (promotes the flow of energy and the storage of energy and blood), and strengthens the *jing* (slows aging).
- *Atractylodes* (*bai zhu, Atractylodes macrocephala rhizome*): bitter,

sweet taste, warm temperature, stabilizes the exterior, benefits the Qi, tonifies the spleen/pancreas, and dries dampness.

- Cinnamon twig (*gui zhi, Cinnamomi ramulus*): acrid, sweet taste, warm temperature, adjusts the protective Qi, warms the channels, disperses cold, moves and strengthens the yang, and transforms Qi.
- *Siler fang feng* (*ledebouriellae sesloidis radix*): acrid, sweet taste, slightly warm temperature, releases the exterior, expels wind cold, and expels wind damp.

Constipation

There are so many ways to treat constipation using Chinese herbs that there are whole categories of herbs devoted to this (see Chapter 7, "Herbs and Their Categories"). However, of all the herbs and their categories, one stands out above the rest: Chinese rhubarb (*da huang, Rhizoma rei*). This herb is used in numerous formulas to treat constipation of various origins.

In Marco Polo's time, the Chinese rhubarb was used for constipation. Chinese rhubarb rhizome (not rhubarb the food) was the most sought-after medicine of its time and a big reason for East-West trade for almost a thousand years.

Run chang wan (*Fructus rersica* teapills, *Rhubarb radix*, or Peach Kernel pill, Moisten Intestines pill) was the first recorded in the *Treatise on the Spleen and Stomach* by Li-Ao in 1249 AD. This herbal blend, which brings out the best qualities of Chinese rhubarb, is safer than senna or other single herb laxatives. It works as a tonic (strengthening) formula with a laxative effect, and is not just a simple purgative. These qualities make it better for long-term use than common laxatives.

Note that when constipation lasts more than a week, it is prudent to consult a physician. Also note that using this or any laxative during pregnancy should be avoided.

Herbal Treatments

Single Herbs, Constituents, and Functions
- Rhubarb rhizome (*da huang, Rhizoma rei*): moves stool, drains heat, invigorates the blood, and detoxifies fire poison.

- Chinese foxglove root (*sheng di huang, Rehmannia glutinosa radix*): nourishes yin and blood, generates fluids, clears heat, and cools blood.
- Ophthipogon tuber (*mai men dong, Ophiopogonis, tuber*): moistens the intestines, nourishes the yin, and clears heat.
- Tang quai root (*dang gui, Angelica sinensis*): tonifies blood, invigorates blood, moistens the intestines, and moves stool.
- Peach seed kernel (*tao ren, Persica semen*): breaks congealed blood, moistens dryness, and lubricates intestines.
- Unripe bitter orange (*zhi ke, Citri immaturus fructus*): directs the Qi downward, moves stool, breaks stagnations, reduces accumulations.

Also available is Bio Essence brand *tong bian wan* (Moving Colon pill), which adds the tonic herb *he shou wu* to the *run chang wan* formula, enhancing its effectiveness for constipation in the elderly or after childbirth. Other useful products for constipation include Aquilaria pills and Aquilaria Stomachic pills. Because they both employ the Qi mover *aloeswood chen xiang* (*Lignum aquilaria*), they are especially good for constipation accompanied by abdominal pain. Both are imported patent medicines made by the Lanzhou Foci herb factory in Lanzhou, China.

In cases of severe constipation or impacted stool, *da huang* can be used alone, unaccompanied by other herbs. It is available in this form as Plum Flower brand Da Huang Jiang Zhi Wan. For more information about this herb, see Chapter 5, "Famous Herbal Medicines."

For those who wish to relieve constipation gently, avoiding purgatives altogether, Plum Flower brand Wu Ren Wan (Five Seed pill) contains no rhubarb or other purgatives. It achieves its laxative effect from the lubricating action of its five oil-bearing seeds.

Cysts and Other Accumulations

Disease Condition Most chronic swellings, including cysts and tumors, are called accumulations, accretions of tissue that build up over time. They occur in the body, as elsewhere in nature, from impediments to flow. Some accumulations, such as cysts, occur because of poor flow combined with an excess of fluids (damp) in the body. Other interior conditions, such as heat, cold, or toxicity, can contribute to the nature of these accumulations.

Cysts are hard to treat because they are closed sacks of fluid, isolated from normal flow of Qi, blood, or other body fluids. This makes them difficult to reach with either Western medicines or Chinese herbs that act through the bloodstream.

Non-Herbal Treatments Qi permeates all the tissue. Acupuncture, which affects the flow of Qi and is not dependent on blood flow, may be helpful for some people in reducing or eliminating cysts and preventing their occurrence. I have had success using acupuncture to treat even bone-hard cysts. Chinese medicine practitioners do not puncture the cysts; needles are placed around the cyst as well as in points downstream along the channels that pass through the area of the growth. Sometimes a small electric stimulator is attached to the needles to stimulate the points.

Big cysts are harder to treat than small ones, and cysts on the interior are more difficult to treat than those on the surface. Occasionally, small cysts in the skin disappear after a single treatment, but it is unlikely that large ovarian cysts would vanish as a result of either acupuncture or herbs.

Herbal Treatments   Several Chinese herbal remedies may be helpful in reducing and preventing the formation of ovarian and other cysts by increasing flow, breaking blood obstructions, dissolving phlegm, and warming interior cold. Recommended formulas are:

- Cysts and tumors: Zedoria tablets, Seven Forests brand
- Breast cysts: Bupleurum Entangled Qi, Health Concerns brand
- Testicular cysts: Ji Shen Ju He Wan (Citrus Seed Pills), several imported brands
- Ovarian cysts: Wen Jing Tang, Herbal Times, Plum Flower, and several other imported brands
- Ovarian cysts: Gui Zhi Fuling san, Herbal Times, Plum Flower, and several imported brands
- Systemic damp: Er Chen Wan, many imported brands
- Neck cysts, goiter, or swollen lymph nodes: Hai Zao Wan, several imported brands
- Tumors: Chih ko and Curcuma, Seven Forest brand

Depression and Anxiety

Disease Condition   Western medicine addresses depression and anxiety as brain problems caused by abnormal brain chemistry. Pharmaceutical drugs alter the brain's chemistry, simulating the feeling of normalcy. In contrast, Chinese medicine understands depression and anxiety as heart problems that are caused by constraint of emotion in the chest. Practitioners believe that changes in brain chemistry are secondary to, and sometimes a consequence of, this emotional constraint.

Loss, memory of loss, repressed expression, and other traumatic events cause constraint in the chest, restraining the normal flows in the central and upper body. This phenomenon is known as Liver Qi Stagnation. Constraint of energy in the chest overstimulates the heart, creating symptoms of anxiety and insomnia. However, sleeplessness is not the worst outcome of stuck Qi in the chest. Difficult conditions such as panic attacks, heart attacks, heart arrhythmias, and even some forms of psychosis have their origins in Liver Qi Stagnation.

Other Treatments   Though drugs are effective in relieving depression, relief can also be obtained by physically freeing the Qi of the chest, which releases this energy. Push-ups work as well as Prozac. Acupuncture helps. Accupuncture points used for depression are on the head, neck, wrists, and chest.

Other ways to release the chest include boxing, breathing exercises, yoga techniques, massage of the chest, shoulder blades, and inner arms, forceful crying and wailing, and almost any upper body exercise. Expressive use of the hands stimulates the channels that nourish the chest, so that activities as varied as gardening, giving massage, swimming the breaststroke, and playing basketball can offer relief. Results from these techniques are instantaneous and can last for hours or days.

Herbal Treatments   Chinese herbs relieve depression and anxiety by moving the liver Qi (Qi of the chest). Taken alone, these herbs may exert only a mild effect. In certain combinations, however, the results can be quite powerful. Hare's Ear Root (*chai hu, Bupleurum*) is

the best known of these herbs. Though it is classified as a surface-re-
lieving herb (used against colds), its most common use is to move the
Qi of the chest. Its ability to do this is greatly enhanced by combining
it with a small amount of mint (*bo he*).

Other Recommended Herbs *He huan pi* (*huan hua*, mimosa bark or
flower, *Albezzia*) is classified as a heart-nourishing herb. This herb, when
combined with *dan shen* (*salvia miltorrhiza*) also strongly moves the Qi
of the chest. Other herbs used in these formulas include poria (*fu shen*),
red dates (*hong zao*), and wheat berries (*fu xiao mai*). Oyster shell (*mu li*),
fossil bone (*long gu*), amber (*hu po*), and loadstone (*ci shi*) are strong stabi-
lizing agents, and are administered for limited periods of time to stabilize
the spirit (see Chapter 5, "Famous Herbal Medicines").

Free and Easy pill (*xiao yao wan*, rambling powder) is a 900-year-
old formula that relieves constraint and promotes the free flow of
Qi in the chest (see "Famous Herbal Medicines"). It is the primary
formula of practitioners when treating depression, but there are alternatives. Variations of *xiao yao wan* such as *jia wei xiao yao wan* also
contain herbs to cool heart fire and/or settle the spirit. Heart Fire and
Restless Spirit (*shen*) are conditions that accompany or complicate
many cases of depression.

Good Sleep and Worry-Free pill, Dr. Shen's brand: nourishes the
heart, calms the spirit, and clears heart fire. Use for anxiety, insomnia,
and restlessness.

Chai hu long gu mu li wan, Plum Flower and other brands: settles
the spirit. Use for palpitations and psychosis.

Emperor's Pills (*tian wang bu xin wan*), many brands available: calms
the spirit, nourishes heart yin. Use for insomnia and mental fatigue.

Diabetes

According to the terminology of Chinese medicine, diabetes is called
the Wasting and Thirsting Disease, caused by a collapse of the yin
of the kidney, the spleen, or the lungs. Research and a great body of
human experience have shown that Chinese herbal medicine can be
helpful for treating type 2 (adult onset) diabetes. For the best results,

it is important to begin with a Chinese medical diagnosis that identifies the organs involved. This enables the practitioner to construct a formula appropriate for the individual pattern. Different herbs and formulas are required to build yin in various organs.

Herbal Treatments   Commonly used formulas are variations of Rehmannia Six (*liu wei di huang*), jade fluid decoction (*yu ye tang*), and Great Yin Tonifying pills (*da bu yin wan*). Other herbs and acupuncture are added to treat complications of diabetes, such as peripheral neuropathy and cataracts.

For patterns involving upper *jiao* with thirst, *yu ye tang* (jade fluid decoction) is a good choice. For patterns involving the middle *jiao* with gnawing hunger or thirst, add *bai hu tang wan* (White Tiger pills) to *liu wei di huang*. For patterns involving the lower *jiao* marked by frequent urination, use *jin gui shen qi wan* (Golden Book pills). For cataracts or eye problems due to diabetes, use *ming mu di huang wan*.

Recommended Single Herbs

- White fungus: (*bai mu er, Fructificatio tremella*)
- Fenugreek seed: (*hu lu ba, Semen trigonella*)
- Trichosianthis root: (*tian hua fen, Radix trichosanthis*)
- American ginseng: (*xi yang shen, Radix panacis quinquifolium*)

Bitter melon (*ku gua, Momordica charantia*), the Asian vegetable, may also be valuable to diabetics. The fresh juice of the unripe bitter melon has been shown to lower blood sugar levels. Three different chemical constituents of this gourd are known to have hypoglycemic (blood sugar lowering) actions beneficial in diabetes.

Diabetes Research Using Chinese Medicine   According to a French study conducted at the Universite Paris-Nord, Hospital Jean-Verdier, France, Chinese herbal medicine offered effective treatment for patients diagnosed with type 2 diabetes. The research can be found in "Randomized Study of Glibenclamide Versus Traditional Chinese Treatment in Type 2 Diabetic Patients," by M.Vray and J. R. Rattali, in *Diabetes et Metabolisme*.

The researchers evaluated the efficacy of a traditional Chinese treatment based on three plants in association with a *sulfonylurea, glibenclamide* (2.5 milligrams three times a day). A randomized double-blind trial was established involving 216 patients in four groups, all of whom were type 2 diabetic outpatients, forty to seventy years of age, being treated by diet alone or by oral anti-diabetic drugs.

Blood tests were used to monitor changes in blood sugar levels. The researchers found that those patients receiving the Chinese medical treatment experienced significantly decreased blood glucose values only two hours after the test meal. Hypoglycemia occurred in nineteen patients in the control groups, but none were recorded in the Chinese herb group. The Chinese plants tested were found to be well tolerated and effective in the treatment of type 2 diabetes.

In another study, a small, randomized clinical trial showed that treatment with American ginseng (*Panax quinquefolius*) helped improve glucose tolerance in non-diabetic people as well as those with type 2 diabetes mellitus. For the study, ten non-diabetic people and nine people with type 2 diabetes received treatment with American ginseng or placebo capsules either forty minutes before or in combination with an oral glucose challenge.

Results showed that in non-diabetic participants, no difference was observed in glycemia between placebo and ginseng when the substances were administered along with glucose, but significant reductions were seen when ginseng was taken forty minutes before the glucose. However, compared with placebo, both ginseng dosage regimens improved glucose tolerance in the people with diabetes.

Information about this study is in *American Ginseng (Panax quinquefolius L.) Reduces Postprandial Glycemia* in "Nondiabetic Subjects and Subjects with Type 2 Diabetes Mellitu," V. Vuksan, J. L. Stevenpiper, V. Y. Y. Koo, et al., in *Archives of Internal Medicine* 160 (2000): 1009–13.

Digestive Problems

Digestion transforms food into Qi and blood that nourish the mind and body. The cycle of hunger and satiety is an underlying rhythm in life, like the heartbeat or the breath. Since irregularity is neither considered good for the heart nor helpful for breathing, it is easy to see that irregularity in eating is bad for digestion and consequently undermines the body's Qi.

The importance of good eating habits, beginning with regularity, cannot be overstated. By recognizing regularly repeating cycles, the body learns to operate efficiently. When food is anticipated, the body prepares itself for digestion. A multitude of activities occur. Enzymes and acids are produced, hormones are activated, thoughts change. When food does not arrive, the entire bodily preparation was a waste of energy, which will have to be repeated again when food finally does arrive. Under these circumstances, it takes twice the energy to digest food. How long can the body drain its systems in this way without consequence? Eventually it will not be able to make enough digestive juices, or will be unable to release them in the proper sequence, resulting in digestive disharmony.

Non-Herbal Treatments Acupuncture and massage can be enormously helpful in dealing with many digestive problems. There is one particularly powerful acupuncture point that is used for the treatment of nausea, indigestion, intestinal pain, and many other digestive complaints. The point is Stomach 36, also known as *zu san li*. Massage and moxibustion (heat treatment) work well on it, so you don't need needles. The point is located on the leg, in a groove about one finger-breadth lateral to the shin and about three inches below the bottom of the kneecap. It is a large point, so you do not need to be right on target to get results. Massage this point deeply for at least five minutes.

Acupuncture can help many digestive conditions. Points are commonly located on the abdomen. Practitioners also use points on the stomach and spleen channels. The digestion segments of these channels are located on the lower leg, usually between the ankle and the knee. The stomach channel runs parallel and lateral to (outside) the tibia (shin bone). The spleen channel runs medially (inside) the shin bone along the calf of the leg.

Although acupuncture is helpful, herbs are often the best medicine for most digestive complaints. Herbs go directly to and through the digestive system. In acute problems, results can be immediate. Chronic digestive problems can be long and complex with many roots and other entanglements. Nevertheless, some life-long problems can be significantly improved or resolved within a few weeks or months.

Herbal Treatments for Heartburn, Reflux, GRD, and Slow Digestion Normally, digestive Qi (energy) flows downward. Heartburn, acid reflux, and gastric reflux diseases are familiar symptoms of abnormal flow. With this condition, also known as Rebellious Stomach Qi, the digestive energy is backing upward instead of flowing downward as it should. This condition can have several root causes that frequently occur in combination.

Western medicine treats these conditions only by suppressing or neutralizing stomach acids. Though this can relieve symptoms, it does not address any of the following possible underlying causes:

- Weak digestive Qi: insufficient digestive enzymes and acids, and weak downward flow of Qi (spleen deficiency).
- Offense to the digestion: such as food poisoning, overeating, undereating, eating difficult-to-digest foods, and irregular or improper eating habits.
- Compulsive thoughts: an event, relationship, memory, or other thought that cannot, figuratively, be swallowed or disgested.
- Hot liver: usually caused by anger or frustration leading to constraint in the chest, which heats the liver and injures the digestion (liver invades stomach).
- Blockage: a physical blockage causes impaired or reversed flow, usually in the intestines (stuck Qi).

Recommended Herbal Medicines by Condition
- Weak digestive Qi: (*xiang sha liu jun zi wan, Aplotaxis amomi pills*): Chinese patent medicine, many brands available
- Overeating: Stomach Curing pills or Po Chai pills, many brands available, both imported and domestic.
- Haw Flakes or Haw Cakes: candy wafers made of hawthorn berries, available at any Asian grocery.

- Emotions injuring digestion: (*Shu Gan Wan*) liver invades stomach, Chinese patent medicine, many brands available
- Intestinal stagnation (constipation): *Rhubarb radix*, Peach Kernel pills, many brands available
- Constraint of chest Qi: Free and Easy pills (*Xiao Yao Wan*), many brands available

Herbs for Diarrhea   Diarrhea is a sign of injury or imbalance to the spleen Qi (digestive energy). This disharmony can generally be seen as yin and yang, though the actual causes are far more numerous.

Hot Diarrhea: Yang Type, Excess Type   Hot type of diarrhea is generally caused by a hot external pathogen such as a virus, bacteria, fungus, or other microorganism. The onset is usually sudden, the odor strong, and may be accompanied by blood in the stool. The pulse is often rapid, and the tongue body may be red, or the coating yellowish. This is typical of dysentery caused by drinking or eating contaminated food. Taking *huang lian su* promptly will usually shorten the course of this ailment.

Cold Diarrhea: Yin Type, Deficient Type   Cold type of diarrhea is usually related to protracted behaviors or deficiencies. It originates from many sources, including emotional patterns such as worry and frustration, poor diet or eating habits, and congenital digestive weakness. In many of these cases, the tongue is characteristically swollen, flabby, or pale. The tongue coating may thicken with internal dampness often consequent to this condition. The onset of this type is usually gradual, characterized by a mild odor and mild and loose stool (with mucous or undigested food).

Long-term use of spleen tonics is recommended for this condition. Spleen Qi must also be conserved. Eating habits should be moderate and regular, and foods should be warm, cooked, and easy to digest. Cold foods, raw foods, and other difficult-to-digest foods should be minimized, as they require too much energy to digest.

Hot and Cold: Yin and Yang Type, Mixed Type   These conditions exhibit both hot and cold symptoms either concurrently or alternately.

Some are diagnosed as inflammatory bowel diseases, such as Crohn's disease or ulcerative colitis. Such conditions are complex, involving cyclical issues of yin turning into yang, and of deficient becoming excess. They can be successfully treated with Chinese herbs, but require experience. Do not attempt self-treatment in these cases.

Ear Problems: Ear Ringing and Hearing Loss

Ringing in the ears (tinnitus) and loss of hearing can share several causes. Some are considered excess in nature, while others are thought of as deficient conditions.

Excess Ear Ringing or Deafness Excess ear ringing (tinnitus) or deafness is caused either by an actual obstruction, like a swelling or a constriction, or an oversupply of Qi. Both result in congestion of fluids. Injury due to loud noise is considered an excess condition. Cysts, scar tissue, or minute swellings within the ear are other examples of excess conditions. The diagnosis of damp heat in the gallbladder channel is commonly associated with the excess type of hearing problems. This diagnosis suggests congestion of fluids and/or infections in the ear. (The gallbladder channel runs through the ear and should not be confused with the actual gallbladder.) This type of hearing loss or ear ringing usually has a sudden onset, and can often be remedied within a week using acupuncture or a strong dose of long *dan xie gan wan*, an excellent formula with a litany of uses. Most herbal medicine manufacturers make a version of this formula.

Deficiency Ear Ringing Deficiency ear ringing (tinnitus), on the other hand, is like the warning buzz that a smoke alarm emits to caution that its batteries are low. The onset of this condition is usually gradual. This type of ear ringing is usually associated with vacuous kidney yin (see The Twelve Organs in Chapter 3, "Understanding Theories of Chinese Medicine"). Treatment is often protracted and best done with supplemental herbs. The herbal medicine used most often is *er ming zuo ci wan* (ear ringing, left [yin] loving pills). This formula combines the formula *liu wei di huang* (see chapter 5, "Famous

Herbal Medicines") with the herbs *Bupleurum* (*chai hu*) and loadstone (*ci shi*) to direct the action to the ears and to settle the rising yang that we perceive as ear ringing. This pill is available from Minshan, Herbal Times, Dr. Shen's, Lanzhou, and several other manufacturers.

Eczema, Psoriasis, and Inflammatory Skin Diseases

Eczema, psoriasis, and other chronic rash-like conditions are all signs of internal heat. Often the Western diagnosis is sufficient to provide a course of treatment with acupuncture or herbs. However, sometimes the diagnosis of eczema or psoriasis does not provide enough information for the practitioner to understanding the source of the heat. Patterns as dissimilar as Toxic Heat in the Blood, Yin Deficiency Heat, Blood Deficiency Dryness, and other syndromes can be diagnosed as either eczema or psoriasis.

Cases where general formulas are unsuccessful will require herbs and acupuncture appropriate to the correct Chinese diagnosis. Resolving these conditions requires understanding the root causes.

Determining the Root Causes   In Chinese Medical theory, there are various kinds of heat. There is heat you can measure, such as a fever, and heat you cannot, such a hot flash. No matter the type or source, heat sets matters in motion and triggers activity. It appears as inflammation, hyperactivity, or over-stimulation. Heat can come from irritating chemicals, foreign organisms, or by the friction caused by the constrained flow of Qi (energy). It is also the by-product of the body's metabolism and digestion. Hormonal activity causes and is stimulated by heat. An overly stimulating diet can cause excess heat, as can a hyperactive mind or lifestyle. Our skin presents the symptoms of heat as rashes, redness, pimples, boils, dryness, infections, and other skin inflammations.

Common sources of heat: overconsumption of stimulating foods, hormonal activity, exertion or physical activity, blood insufficient to dilute toxins, agitated thoughts, atmospheric heat (hot weather), constraint of Qi, and blood stagnation.

Eczema Sometimes heat is caused by blood deficiency. When blood is deficient, it can cause more problems than just dryness. Deficient blood cannot properly dilute normal cell wastes (toxins) that must be transported in the blood. Toxic heat in the blood will result. This condition will be diagnosed as many different inflammatory skin diseases. Eczema is often diagnosed when internal heat generates dryness in the skin.

Dryness can come from heat, fluid deficiency, or a dry environment. Dry weather, wind, or the influence of drying substances can cause internal and external dryness. Dryness can also come from deficiency of blood or other fluids. Internal heat, whether from feverish disease or from fluid deficiency, will further scorch the fluids and cause more dryness.

Herbal Treatments for Eczema Use this formula alone or add herbs for different kinds of eczema:

Jing jie, six grams	*Zhi mu*, six grams
Fang feng, six grams	*Sheng di huang*, six grams
Niu bang zi, six grams	*Shi gao*, six grams
Chan tui, three grams	*Mu dan pi*, six grams
Yi yi ren, six grams	*Gan cao*, three grams

For itching, add *ku shen*, six grams
For skin dryness, add *mai men dong*, six grams
For scalp eczema, add *huang qin and chuan xiong*, six grams
For ear eczema, add *long dan cao*, six grams
For elbow, knee, and other joint related eczema, add *bai shao*, six grams
For blood deficiency, add Eight Treasures (Women's Precious pills), twelve grams
For stress-induced heat, add Free and Easy pills or *Jia Wei Xiao Yao Wan*, twelve grams

Psoriasis Psoriasis (*song pi xian*) is not simply a topical condition. It is rooted in internal dryness. Chinese herbal medicine can help most sufferers with this condition. When it appears in dotted form, it is called *bai bi* and is caused by undernourishment of the skin due to blood dryness. Such dryness can be caused by invasion of pathogenic wind or by heat. There are three kinds of psoriasis:

Psoriasis caused by flaming of heat-evil combined with wind Symptoms: erythema (red spots or blotches) and scales appear, spreading throughout the skin. The lesions are usually red and raised. The scales flake off easily when scratched. Itching can be severe. Use Cool the Blood and Expel Wind (*liang xue xiao feng tang*). Ingredients:

> *Sheng di huang (Radix rehmanniae glutinosae);* thirty grams
> *Sheng shi gao (gypsum):* fifteen grams
> *Bai mao gen (Rhizoma imperatae cylindricae):* thirty grams
> *Xuan shen (Radix scrophulariae ningpoensis):* nine grams
> *Zhi mu (Radix anemarrhenae asphodeloidis):* twelve grams
> *Bai shao (Radix paeoniae lactiflorae):* nine grams
> *Jin yin hua (Flos lonicerae japonicae):* fifteen grams
> *Niu bang zi (Fructus arctii lappae):* nine grams
> *Jing jie (Herba seu flos schizonepetae tenuifoliae):* nine grams
> *Fang feng (Radix ledebouriellae sesloidis):* nine grams
> *Gan cao (Radix glycyrrhizae uralensis):* nine grams

Psoriasis caused by blood-heat and stasis Symptoms: The lesions and swellings are less severe than in the previous condition. New lesions, which appear only sporadically, are usually purple-red and may be covered by a thick layer of scales. Use the formula *niu pi xuan hao fang*. Ingredients:

> *Tu fu ling (Rhizoma smilacis glabrae):* thirty grams
> *Sheng di huang (Radix rehmanniae glutinosae):* thirty grams
> *Ban lan gen (Radix isatidis seu baphicacanthin):* fifteen grams
> *Da Qing ye (Folium daqingye):* fifteen grams
> *Xuan shen (Radix scrophulariae ningpoensis):* nine grams
> *Mai men dong (Tuber ophiopogonis japonici):* nine grams
> *Jin yin hua (Flos lonicerae japonicae):* nine grams
> *Lian Qiao (Fructus forsythiae suspensae):* nine grams
> *Huang Qin (Radix scutellariae baicalensis):* nine grams
> *Dang gui (Radix angelicae sinensis):* nine grams
> *Hong hua (Flos carthami tinctorii):* nine grams

Psoriasis caused by toxic-heat and blood-stasis Symptoms: The lesions are dark red or pigmented and covered by thick, hard scales that do not flake off. Sometimes lesions overlap, causing the skin to take on a map-like appearance. They itch, hurt, or fissure. In other cases, the joints are affected. These lesions can persist for years. Use the formula *niu pi xuan er hao fang*. Ingredients:

Tu fu ling (Rhizoma smilacis glabrae): thirty grams
Yin chen hao (Herba artemisiae capillaris): fifteen grams
Sheng di huang (Radix rehmanniae glutinosae): fifteen grams
Jin yin hua (Flos lonicerae japonicae): fifteen grams
Lian qiao (Fructus forsythiae suspensae): fifteen grams
Sheng shi gao (gypsum): fifteen grams
Pu gong ying (Herba taraxaci mongolici cum radice): ten grams
Zi hua di ding (Herba violae cum radice): ten grams
San leng (Rhizoma sparganii): ten grams
Ye ju hua (Flos chrysanthemi indici): ten grams

External Treatments for Psoriasis

Ointment *(pu lian gao)*. Ingredients:

Huang qin (Radix scutellariae baicalensis): fifty grams
Huang bai (Cortex phellodendri): fifty grams
Vaseline: 400 grams

Method: Grind the first two herbal ingredients into fine powder and make an ointment by mixing the powder with Vaseline.

Bathe in a decoction Ingredients:
Ku shen (Radix sophorae flavescentis): sixty grams
Tu fu ling (Rhizoma smilacis glabrae): thirty grams
Yin chen hao (Herba artemisiae capillaris): thirty grams
Da huang (Rhizoma rhei): thirty grams
Ye ju hua (Flos chrysanthemi indici): thirty grams
Zi hua di ding (Herba violae cum radice): thirty grams
Gan cao (Radix glycyrrhizae uralensis): thirty grams

Method: Immerse in the bath daily for thirty to forty minutes.

Energy Issues and Chronic Fatigue

Non-Herbal Treatments Chinese medicine offers a unique and often highly successful approach to ailments that leave a person with low energy. The disciplines of Qi Gong and Tai Chi deal with the cultivation of energy and how these energies are used to improve health. Since energy (Qi) must move after it has been cultivated, all modalities require moving the Qi as part of the process of dealing with it once built up. Acupuncture can also help.

Chinese medicine is all about energy. Each person is a universe of energies with complex qualities, production, and distribution components. Therefore, treating symptoms of low energy using Chinese medicine is rarely simple. Westerners tend to seek magic drugs or herbs that will restore lost energy, or pump up the muscles in order to excel, compete, or exceed normal limits. Every year a new energy herb is touted as the next wonder drug. Many of these are Chinese herbs. Ginseng, goji berries, *fo ti*, cordyceps, *jiao gu lan, Astragalus*, and others have held the spotlight. Though these are wonderful herbs, none of them are a universal cure for low energy.

Curing energy problems that have symptoms of malaise, fatigue, or exhaustion requires a diagnosis of the underlying disharmonies. Moreover, multiple conditions usually underlie chronic symptoms. People with chronic fatigue should consult an experienced Chinese herbologist.

However, when you are without access to professional help, and you can attempt a simple diagnosis, you can use or combine the following herbal products. They have been selected because they will do little or no harm if your diagnosis is incorrect and they are taken inappropriately. Most of these remedies are also mentioned in Chapter 5, "Famous Herbal Medicines."

Disease Condition and Herbal Treatments

Spleen Qi Deficiency Symptoms: Fatigue with digestive complaints such as gas, bloating, loose stool; fatigue after eating; muscle weakness. Remedy: Six Gentlemen pills (see Chapter 5, "Famous Herbal Medicines").

Kidney Deficiency Symptoms: Fatigue with lower back pain, weak knees, or low libido; waking up tired after normal sleep; loss of hearing or ringing in the ears (tinnitus). Remedy: Golden Book pills or other variant of *liu wei di huang*.

Prolonged Viral Disease Symptoms: Fatigue with fever, body aches; positive test results for viral presence. Remedy: Combine *gan mao ling* with *zong gan ling* (see Cold and Flu section of this chapter).

Blood Deficiency Symptoms: Weak and tired, especially after menses; menstrual problems such as irregular periods, light flow, headaches after menses; poor concentration; skin problem. Remedy: Women's Precious pills.

Menopause and Yin Deficiencies Symptoms: Feeling tired or exhausted; experiencing night sweats, afternoon fevers, or hot flashes; dry skin, eyes, and/or hair; reduced vaginal fluids, reduced ejaculate, low libido. Remedy: Two Immortals pills and/or *Zhi Bai Di Huang Wan* (see "Famous Herbal Medicines").

Epilepsy and Seizures

Epilepsy is a disharmony characterized by unprovoked seizures. In Chinese medical terminology, it is called seizure disorder. Several different causes underly this disease; they must be diagnosed before the disease can be treated.

First, epilepsy can be caused by trauma to the brain. Before any further diagnosis can be made, brain damage should be either confirmed or ruled out. This diagnosis is made by history, physical examination, brain scans, and other modern medical techniques. Modern techniques are essential to accurately detect brain damage and must be employed.

Non-Herbal Treatments When brain damage is found, scalp acupuncture is reported to be an effective treatment. Scalp acupuncture is used to treat a variety of brain diseases, including hemiplegia and aphasia following stroke, as well as other symptoms of brain damage. Rather than inserted perpendicularly as in most other instances, fine needles are threaded parallel to, and just under, regions of the scalp that cover affected areas of the brain. Needles are often rotated quickly or stimulated with electricity. Done correctly, this will not hurt, but few acupuncturists are versed in this technique. You might want to ask your acupuncturist about his or her experience with scalp acupuncture before undergoing treatment.

Herbal Treatments When brain damage is the cause of epilepsy, herbs for injury and herbs for brain function are given together. Remedy: Ching Koo pills (contraindicated for pregnancy). A Chinese patent medicine for injury, it can be combined with any *bu nao* (tonify brain) formula. Either Cerebral Tonic pills or Healthy Brain pills will do. Several brands are available wherever Chinese medicines are sold. You may want to avoid the Bu Nao brand formula, also known as An Sen Pu Naw, made by Chung Lien Drug Works, because it lists cinnabar (mercuric sulfide) as one of its ingredients.

When brain damage is not the cause of epilepsy, seizures are usually related to Internal Wind, and will fall into two distinct types, which will dictate the treatment protocol. To know which seizure is which, one must be able to tell yin from yang.

Yin Seizures and Yang Seizures All seizures, from a Traditional Chinese Medicine point of view, are caused by Internal Wind. Fainting, strokes, seizures, childhood convulsions, paralysis, palsy, and even facial tics are attributed to Internal Wind.

Yin Seizures, Open Seizures Yin seizures, also known as open seizures or Wei Syndrome, are marked by open or flaccid paralysis. Passing out, going limp, and fainting are yin seizures. Yin seizures are most often caused by underlying deficiency, but may also be caused by phlegm obstructions preventing the normal flow of Qi and blood to the head (as in a stroke). Wei Syndrome can include symptoms of muscular weakness, atrophy, trembling, tingling, or numbness. Modern diagnosis of sequelae to stroke, ALS, myasthenia gravis, Parkinson's disease, polio, and Guillain Barre disease all indicate possible Wei Syndrome.

Remedy: Tian Ma Mi Huan tablets There are several brands of this medicine, all of which combine gastrodia (*tian ma*) with honey mushroom (*mi huan jun, Armillaria*). These two herbs grow together underground. Both have tonic properties. *Tian ma* prevents internal wind and is said to stimulate blood circulation to the brain and heart. *Mi huan jun* is said to also improve circulation to the brain and extremities.

Remedy: Zai zao wan There are many brands and versions of this medicine available. All contain some variation of the term *zai zao (tsai tsao, jai jao)*, meaning "restorative." All are appropriate for open seizures, and are most often used following a stroke. Do not use this herb during pregnancy.

Yang Seizures, Closed Seizures Yang seizures, on the other hand, are clenched, spastic, or rigid, and are called closed seizures. Liver wind causes most closed seizures. Liver wind is stirred up by liver fire, which in turn can be set ablaze by any number of provocations. The liver tends to run hot. Emotions, environmental influences, and deficiencies are all capable of overheating the liver. Even systemic imbalances outside the liver can affect it. Though liver wind is considered excess in nature, sometimes the pattern is caused by a lack of yin fluids that normally cool the hot liver. In other cases, overexposure to toxic chemicals can overwork the liver. The most frequent cause is emotional constraint, which can bind and overheat the liver, also resulting in Internal Wind.

The following herbal medicines can be used when epilepsy is a sign of Excess Liver Yang and Wind. They are also used to treat high blood pressure, which in itself is a sign of Liver Wind. Most of these formulas are old, well established, and easy to find.

Bupleurum and dragon bone: *chai hu long gu muli wan*
Sedate Liver pill: *jiang ya wan*
Compound cortex eucommia pill: *fu fang* du zhong pian*
Hypertension repressing tablets: *jiang ya ping pian*
* The term fu fang means "medicinal compound" and occasionally indicates that herbs have been compounded with drugs or other supplements, though probably not in this particular case.

Hair Loss and Prematurely Gray Hair

The story is that long ago, an old man, Mr. He, became lost in the forest, where he ate only the root of a common vine. Years later, when he was reunited with his tribe, those who found him were astonished. The old man's hair had turned from white to black. After returning to his clan, he is said to have fathered two more children. Today the root bears his name, Old Mr. He (*he shou wu*). In the West, it is known as fleece flower root, *Polygoni multiflori,* or *fo ti.* Modern practitioners of Chinese medicine use this herb to strengthen the blood and the *jing* to treat alopecia, prevent premature hair loss and graying, and to regulate excessive aging.

Disease Condition

Hair Loss Healthy hair depends on an abundant flow of Qi and blood to the scalp and hair roots. When this nourishing flow is compromised, the hair will suffer. Diminished nourishment is most usually caused by:

- Blood Deficiency. Blood is made through the digestive process, and blood deficiency can be caused by dietary or digestive insufficiencies. Alopecia and other kinds of hair loss can result when the blood lacks these nourishing components.

- Constrained flow (Qi stagnation). Stress and emotional constraint can restrict the flow of Qi and blood in the neck, shoulders, face, and head. Acupuncture, massage, meditation, and relaxation techniques can help restore this flow. Acupuncture and massage may include points on the outsides of the forearms, ankles, feet, neck, shoulders, face, and scalp.

- Patency of the vessels. The size, diameter, and health of the tiny blood vessels that conduct nourishment to the hair can also play a part. Genetic factors as well as acquired factors can affect the patency of the vessels, making these capillaries fragile or narrow.

Gray Hair Premature graying is caused by a deficiency of *jing. Jing* is the substance, energy, program, process, or stuff that affects the course of maturation and aging. When *jing* is weak, one ages rapidly. When *jing* is restored, one becomes vital and mature more slowly.

Herbal Treatment Several herbs appear to reduce aging or restore youthfulness, and are thus considered *jing* tonics. Ginseng is the best known. Among them, *he shou wu* is thought to be best at restoring hair color and reducing hair loss. Though the herb is classified as a blood tonic, it has many other wonderful qualities (see "Herbs that Regulate Blood" in Chapter 7).

Fleece Flower Root (*he shou wu, Polygoni multiflori, fo ti*)

Clinical Functions Strengthens the liver and kidneys, benefits the hair, nourishes the blood, benefits and retains the essence, detoxifies fire poison, moistens the intestines, expels wind from the skin.

Functions according to Chinese medicine: bitter, sweet, astringent taste; slightly warm temperature.

Part of Plant Used root

Indications for Use Thinning or prematurely gray hair; dry, brittle, or damaged hair; excessive or premature aging.

Daily Dosage and Administration Boiled: nine to fifty grams; powder or tablet: one to ten grams.

Course of Use three or more weeks

Headaches

Non-Herbal Treatments Acupuncture is often effective in treating some kinds of headaches. Local points on the head or face, in the area of pain, might or might not be used. Points on the hands, feet, or the base of the spine, however, are almost always chosen to relieve headaches. These points are selected on the distal ends of channels that pass through the painful area on the head. The aim of treatment is to drain the stagnant Qi away from the head and towards the extremities. This technique is successful and employed for headaches diagnosed as "excess" in nature. Headaches diagnosed as stemming from deficiencies of Qi and blood generally respond less well to acupuncture, and must be treated with herbs.

To best treat headaches with acupuncture or Chinese herbs, practitioners use the Four Examinations to diagnose the underlying problem. Modern diagnoses, such as migraine, cluster, stress, or vascular headaches, do not reveal the real causes. A diagnosis through the eyes of Chinese medicine practitioners, however, provides an understanding of the causes and points to the cure.

Disease Condition and Herbal Treatments Headaches fall into two general categories: excess headaches and deficiency headaches. Both result in diminished flow of Qi and blood to the head. This poor flow is experienced as pain.

Excess headaches are caused by an overabundance of Qi and/or blood in the upper body that result in congested or stuck flow in or to the head. This kind of headache could be caused by a concussive injury or by an oversupply of Qi in the upper body. This oversupply can be due to constraint and tension in the head and neck from stressful thoughts, or from heat energy rising in the body. Strong emotions, drugs, toxins, ingesting alcohol, or even eating spicy foods can create heat that will rise to the head and cause a headache.

Deficiency headaches, from deficiency of blood and Qi, result in poor circulation in or to the head. Headaches with weakness or tiredness, or headaches associated with menstrual periods, happen when the head is undernourished by blood or Qi. These headaches are usually chronic and recurrent. They are often accompanied by fatigue, and may get worse before or after menses, when blood is being used in the mansion or blood (lower abdomen) and there is less available for the head. Long-term use of Women's Precious pills (Eight Treasures) is recommended together with the patent medicine *chuan xiong chai ta wan.*

Often, a thorough diagnostic analysis is unnecessary to understand the source of a headache. You can make a pretty good guess about the nature of a headache from its location. This will lead you to the correct remedy most of the time.

One-sided headaches, pain behind the eyes, and pain at the top of the head are called Liver/Gallbladder headaches. They are caused by liver heat rising up the gallbladder channel. Heat generated by anger, frustration, or toxicity will rise along the liver channel and affect the eyes or the head. Heat may easily diverge to the gallbladder channel, affecting the side of the head. Usually a one-sided or migraine headache is considered a Liver/Gallbladder headache. This condition sometimes includes chronic neck and shoulder tension as well. Two popular herbs for this kind of headache are *tian ma gouteng wan* and *long dan xie gan wan.*

Forehead, nose, and cheek pain headaches are usually sinus headaches. Damp accumulations in the head produce swollen tissue, pressure, and painful frontal headaches that are generally unrelieved by conventional anti-inflammatory drugs. Damp conditions also provide a breeding ground for many microorganisms. This condition can result in sinus infections. For sinus headaches, try Dr. Shen's Sinus and Nose pills or the patent medicine *pe min kan wan*.

Frontal headaches, facial pain, and toothache have their source in digestive stagnation. Stomach Fire Headache is caused by heat rising up the stomach channel, which affects the front of the head or face. Headaches associated with nausea, toothache, or painful gums often fall into this category. Most often caused by food stagnation, stomach fire comes from overindulgence, eating at bedtime, overconsumption of spicy food, and other poor eating habits.

Hangover headaches are similar and are caused by a combination of liver and stomach excess. Stomach fire can be quickly cured with White Tiger pills, a Chinese patent medicine. Hangover headaches often yield to Stomach Curing pills.

Whole Head Headaches (Wind Cold, Wind Heat, Wind Damp), considered wind-caused headaches, are due to an invasion from outside the body, like a cold, flu, or overexposure to the elements. Here the wind enters the surface of the upper body and obstructs the normal flow of Qi in the skin and muscle layers, causing pain. These headaches accompany colds, flu, or other diseases caused by airborne organisms. These headaches are commonly associated with the urinary bladder channel, which affects the back of the head in the occipital region. The Chinese patent formula *chuan xiong chai ta wan* is often used for this condition, as is *zong gan ling*, made by Dr. Shen's, Plum Flower, and Herbal Times.

Heart Health

Disease Condition Traditional Chinese Medicine regards the pumping action of the heart and the circulatory system as the yang aspect of the heart. The heart system includes the vessels (*luo*) and the tributaries (*jing luo*). It also includes the electrical energy that triggers the heart to contract (heart Qi).

Heart yin, on the other hand, refers to the emotional aspect of the heart. Terms like "heart and soul," "brave heart," and "heartless" are about the yin of the heart. According to modern medicine, feelings and emotions are brain phenomena not directly related to the heart function. To practitioners of Chinese medicine, however, yin and yang are always related, and a healthy heart yang strongly influences emotions, mind, and spirit.

The heart is home to the *shen*. *Shen* can mean spirit, mind, or supreme being. Conditions of normalcy, including sufficient fluids (heart yin and blood), are needed for the *shen* to be comfortable. When the *shen* is at home in your heart, you feel grounded and centered, and your actions are appropriate and correct. Herbs that build heart blood include longan fruit (*long yan rou*), jujube fruit (*da zao*), and cooked rehmannia root (*shu di huang*).

Deficient heart blood or heart yin can result in Restless Shen, causing irritability, anxiety, or insomnia. Heart palpitations, rapid heartbeat (tacycardia), loss of memory or concentration, and panic disorder also arise from this condition. Two good formulas for heart yin deficiency are Dr. Shen's Good Sleep and Worry-Free pills and Emperor's Tea (*tian huang bu xin tang*).

Other Treatments Regular moderate exercise nourishes the heart by opening the vessels and keeping them flowing. Choose your form of exercise, but practice it between two to five days per week. Too much or too little exercise can cause injury. During exercise, do your best to breathe exclusively through your nose unless your nasal passages are obstructed. Breathing through the mouth permits overexertion, which could overtax the heart or the Qi.

Endeavor to do more, but stop short of your limits. The important part is regularity. Push your limits only occasionally. The martial arts disciplines of Qi Gong and Tai Chi have also been shown to improve heart health.

Herbal Treatments

Weak Heart Deficient heart Qi, coronary insufficiency, heart failure
- Golden Book pill: many brands available (see Chapter 5, "Famous Herbal Medicines")

- *Hai ma bu shen wan:* patent medicine, several brands available
- Pseudoginseng (*tien qi*): a single herb

High Cholesterol Phlegm in the channels, clogged arteries, high cholesterol
- Good Heart pills: Dr. Shen's
- Hawthorn Fat Reducing pills: San Ming Factory, Fujan, China
- *Shan sha jiang zhi wan*: Herbal Times
- Mao Dung Ching pills: Kwangchow Pharmaceutical, Guangzhou, China

Heart Attack/Stroke Heart blood stagnation, angina, heart attack
- Dan shen tablets: patent medicine, several brands available
- Styrax 14 pills: Seven Forest

Excess Emotions Liver attacking heart, stress- or depression-related
- Free and Easy pills: Dr. Shen's and many other brands available

Hepatitis

Disease Condition All types of hepatitis are caused by heat toxins and are known as Damp or Toxic Heat in the Liver and Spleen. The term heat toxin usually refers to viral diseases, but may also include some bacterial infections. Diagnosis determines the proportions of dampness and heat, and the degree of involvement of each organ.

Herbal Treatments Herbs such as *Artemesia capillaris* (*yin chen*), dandelion (*pu gong yin*), atractylodes (*cang zhu*), gardenia seed (*zhi zi*), and bupleurum (*chai hu*) are used to cool and dredge the liver. Liver tonics such as cooked rehmannia (*shu di huang*), white peony (*bai shao*), and eclipta (*han lian cao*) are frequently added to nourish the liver.

Acute Hepatitis Heat toxin formulas (anti-viral)
- *Chuan xin lian* (*Andrographis*): also used for cold and flu, available from United, Plum Flower, and Guangdong brands
- *Gan Mao Tui Re Chong Ji*, also known as *Ban Lan Gen* Tea: also used for cold and flu, several imported brands available at Chinese herb stores

Acute Attack with Pain
- Hepatoplex: Health Concerns brand
- *To jing wan*: also used for pain of menstrual cramps, China National Chemicals, Hangzhou, China

High Fever
- White Tiger pills (*bai hu tang*): Plum Flower

Chronic Hepatitis
- Ecliptex: Health Concerns brand
- Eclipta tablets: Seven Forest brand
- Hepatoplex 1: Health Concerns brand
- *Xiao chai hu tang wan*: Chinese patent medicine, Lanzhou, Plum Flower, and others

Jaundice
- *Yin zhi huang* formula ingredients: *Yin chen* (*Artemesia capillaris*), *zhi zi* (*Gardenia fructus*), and *da huang* (*Rei rhizome*)

Hemorrhoids

Disease Condition Three conditions cause hemorrhoids:
1. Stagnation and heat in the large intestine. This is caused by chronic constipation or by the over-consumption of spicy or stimulating foods (see Foods as Medicines in the appendices).
2. Prolapse of Qi (energy loses its lifting quality). This can happen when the spleen yang Qi is weak or damaged from sudden or prolonged digestive illness, pregnancy, or childbirth. The herbal medicine *bu zhong yi qi wan* (central Qi strengthening pill) is often used for this condition. Many brands are available.
3. Gravity. This is caused by prolonged sitting or standing, walking too long while carrying heavy objects, or reading on the toilet.

Acupuncture can be beneficial for many cases of hemorrhoids, but is seldom a cure. The major points used are at the top of the head; secondary points are at the base of the spine, the hands, and the back of the calves.

Any treatment plan for hemorrhoids must include diagnosing which of the three causes is to be addressed. When heat or stagnation in the intestines is a problem, practitioners need to know the cause. Common reasons include depletion of fluids, an excessively stimulating diet, poor eating habits, constipation, heat pathogens, and emotional constraints.

Herbal Treatments Fargelin pills: There are several variations of this extremely effective formula. Unfortunately, the most effective of them contain much more arsenic than you should take, even for short durations. The Plum Flower version is arsenic-free. Not for children, pregnant women, or nursing mothers.

Topical relief can be obtained by Musk Hemorrhoid Ointment, which contains no musk, or by Bear Gallbladder Ointment, which contains no bear gallbladder. Both feel extremely cold, or may burn for a moment when first applied, so be prepared.

High Blood Pressure (Hypertension)

Disease Condition In English there are two names for this condition: hypertension and high blood pressure. Chinese medical terminology does not have equivalent names. Practitioners of Traditional Chinese Medicine instead investigate the Liver Yang Rising, its signs, symptoms, and consequences, one of which is hypertension.

Hypertension is a consequence of a family of conditions known as liver excess conditions. In increasing order of severity they are: Liver Yang Rising, Liver Heat Rising, Liver Fire Blazing Upward, Interior Liver Wind, and Windstroke. Symptoms of this pattern include headaches, ear ringing, dizziness, vertigo, eye pain, neck and shoulder tension, temporomandibular joint (TMJ) syndrome, or hypertension. These may appear alone, in combination, and in any chronological order.

Although these conditions are considered excess in nature, sometimes the pattern is caused by deficient yin of the liver or kidney. In other cases, emotional constraint can lead to the liver overheating, resulting in excess liver patterns. For this reason, prepackaged herbal patent medicines for hypertension may contain additional herbs to build liver yin or to combat liver Qi stagnation. For those who do not have access to professional help, the following herbs and herbal medicines are considered helpful.

Herbal Treatments to Decrease Blood Pressure

Jiang ya pian (Lower Blood Pressure pills). There are many brands and versions; all combine herbs to nourish the yin with herbs to subdue the yang. Avoid the version known as *chiang ya wan* from Beijing; it contains excessive arsenic and mercury.

Compound Cortex Eucommia pills. These are made by Kweichow United Pharmaceutical in Guizhou, and by Plum Flower. Both are safe and both use the herb *du zhong* (*Eucommia*) as their main ingredient for lowering blood pressure.

Beware of Seven Flower extract, sold online as a Chinese herbal remedy for high blood pressure. Reportedly, it is an unapproved pharmaceutical drug falsely sold as a Chinese herbal medicine.

Herbal Treatments to Increase Blood Pressure

Only a few Chinese herbs are known to increase blood pressure. These are *ma huang* (*Ephedra sinensis*), *gan cao* (licorice), and *ren shen* (ginseng). *Ma huang* has a chemical constituent—ephedrine—that can raise blood pressure. Ephedrine has been removed from most consumer products and is strictly controlled by government authorities. This is largely due to its dangerous overuse as a stimulant and weight-loss product. Licorice can cause hypertension when used in very large doses. Its glycyrrhizin acid component can increase the sodium content of blood, and thus gradually increase blood pressure. It is rare to have such a reaction from normal doses of licorice in Chinese herb formulas.

Ginseng actually has been shown to lower blood pressure at normal dosages (three to four grams per day). Extremely large doses (thirty grams or more per day), however, can raise blood pressure dramatically. It is used in China to treat sudden drops of blood pressure. This should not deter anyone from using ginseng at normal doses.

In addition to ephedra, licorice, and ginseng, the following herbs are suspected of containing alkaloids that might raise blood pressure: aniseed, St. John's wort, capsicum, parsley, blue cohosh, vervain, chaste berry, bayberry, ginger, pau d'arco, coltsfoot, gentian, cola, scotch broom, calamus, and guarana. This does not mean that these herbs cause hypertension. It means only that they contain chemical constituents that might cause blood pressure to rise. As these constituents are only part of an herb's chemical make up, it is unlikely that taking them in traditional dosages will affect blood pressure.

Immunity

The concept of an immune system is relatively recent in the West. In China, doctors have been strengthening the defensive energy (*wei Qi*) for thousands of years. They already understood the concepts of Qi (energy), and of yin and yang (offense and defense). They also knew that Qi could influence our health and be affected by the body's health. They determined that deficiencies of the spleen, lung, or kidney lead to deficient protective energy (*wei Qi*).

Herbal Treatments   The most famous herb for immunity is milk vetch root (*huang Qi*), also known as *Astragalus*. In the *Essentials of the Materia Medica* (1694 AD), it was called "the senior of all herbs." It tonifies the spleen, stomach, Qi, and blood, and benefits the *Wei Qi* (immune system). Research has shown that it can also lower blood pressure and increase endurance. This herb is recognized for increasing the body's resistance and is now considered one of the world's greatest immune tonics.

You can purchase and use this herb alone or in several prepared combinations (see Chapter 5, "Famous Herbal Medicines").
- Jade Windscreen pills (*yu ping feng wan*): several brands available
- Jade Shield pills: Dr. Shen's (similar to Jade Windscreen pills, but may be more suitable for use by dry or yin-deficient people)
- Ginseng Astragalus pill (*Shen Qi wan*); Minshan and Lanzhou brands, Lanzhou, China

Infertility, Pregnancy, and Miscarriage

Infertility   Chinese medicine has long been used to aid fertility. Chinese records on treatment of infertility and miscarriage date back to 200 AD. The first book on gynecology is *The Complete Book of Effective Prescriptions for Diseases of Women*, 1237 AD.

Today in China, acupuncture and herbs are used to treat infertility in both men and women. Clinical trials are regularly reported in Chinese medical journals. Combining Western medical techniques with Chinese methods is common. Some doctors are trained in both methods. Most cases of infertility successfully treated in China are the result of traditional methods, and not the result of modern techniques such as in vitro fertilization (IVF). The Chinese consider modern techniques overly expensive and only modestly successful.

Men are a factor in infertility about 40 percent of the time. Male infertility is usually caused by deficiencies of kidney yang or *jing*. Remedies known as Man's Treasure pills or *nan bao* are widely available everywhere Chinese herbs are sold (see the Sexual Problems section of this chapter).

The herbs used for infertility in men or in women are entirely safe, but, like any food, could on rare occasion cause digestive reactions. This is usually corrected by a modification of the formula or by changing the method of administration. Allergic reactions are extremely rare. Acupuncture treatment is even safer, showing virtually no instances of adverse reactions.

The aim of treatment is to harmonize imbalances to restore normal physiological functions. Treatment can include acupuncture, herbs, movement, meditation, and massage. Treatment aims to restore harmony and balance and eliminate other impediments to conception. As these conditions vary greatly from person to person, treatment protocols will also vary.

Success depends on diagnosing the root disharmonies and then providing correct therapy. Diagnosis is performed according to the Four Examinations (see Chapter 3, "Understanding Theories of Chinese Medicine"). A combination of one or more of the following three patterns is the root of many fertility problems.

Deficiency Pattern A deficiency pattern affects the hormonal system, impairing sexual and reproductive functions, and is usually accompanied by fatigue, a pale tongue, or a weak pulse. Remedies include Dr. Shen's Women's Precious Pills and *nu ke ba zhen wan* made by Lanzhou, Plum Flower, Herbal Times, and others.

Stagnation Pattern A stagnation pattern has the effect of restricting circulation of Qi and blood to the reproductive organs. Acupuncture is the method of choice for stagnation patterns. However, numerous acupuncture points, particularly those on the abdomen and lower back, must be avoided immediately following conception so as not to dislodge a possibly implanted embryo. Herbal medicines include *shao fu zhu yu wan* (stasis in the lower palace pills) and *tao hong si wu tang wan* (*tao ren, persica* and *hong hua, carthamus*), Four Substances pills, both from Plum Flower.

Heat or Cold Pattern A heat or cold pattern causes the affected organs to function abnormally by raising or lowering the local temperature. Remedies include *wen jing tang wan* (Warm the Menses pill) by Plum Flower, and *nuan gong yun zi wan* (Warm the Palace Pregnancy Seed pill) and *fu ke zhong zi wan* (Ova-Seed pill), both by Lanzhou Foci.

A hidden advantage of addressing root problems is that other unintended health benefits can accrue. Regardless of achieving pregnancy, many patients report improvements their health and sense of well being.

As with all medicines, there are no guarantees of success. However, clinical studies in China have shown that 70 percent of all cases of infertility treated by Chinese medicine resulted in pregnancy. Depending on the particular study and the types of infertility treated, success rates ranged from about 50 percent to more than 90 percent.

Notes on In Vitro Fertilization (IVF) Acupuncture and Chinese herbal medicine are valuable complements to in vitro fertilization, and may significantly benefit the outcome of this procedure. According to Dr. Lifang Liang, who conducted experiments using Chinese medicine as an adjunct to IVF at the University of Texas, Chinese medicine increases the success rate of in vitro fertilization by as much as 50 percent. IVF patients are given herbs and acupuncture at several critical stages during the procedure. At the first stage, when birth control pills are administered to regulate hormonal activity, herbs and acupuncture are used to insure the smooth flow of Qi to the ovaries. Next, when drugs are given to stimulate egg production, Chinese herbs and acupuncture are used to ease the stimulating side effects of the drugs. Similar herbs also are used before implantation to relax the muscles, prevent contraction, and better enable the embryo to implant in the uterus.

Other herbs with a long history of preventing miscarriage are used after transfer to strengthen the womb and avert miscarriage.

Miscarriage and Pregnancy

Disease Condition   Once pregnancy is confirmed, treatment is usually discontinued. Only those with a history of miscarriage or those who suffer morning sickness will take herbs or acupuncture during pregnancy. Morning sickness, to practitioners of Chinese medicine, is a possible sign of threatened miscarriage. Chinese medicine can prevent or even stop miscarriage. Dr. Shen's practice has witnessed this many times. When faced with a threatened miscarriage, see an experienced Chinese herbalist immediately. Women with a history of miscarriage should see a Chinese herbologist before attempting conception.

Herbal Treatments

Shi San Tai Pao Wan (Thirteen Weeks Great Protecting pill): use in the first trimester to settle morning sickness, boost energy, and prevent miscarriage. Made by Tianjin in China.

An Tai Wan (Peaceful Fetus pill): use for restless fetus with accumulating heat marked by spotting of blood, cramps, or lower back pain. Use also to ease premature uterine contractions. Made by United Pharmaceutical in Guangzhou.

Specific Causes of Miscarriage and Their Herbal Treatments

Cause   deficiency with stagnation. The flow of nourishment to the fetus is insufficient due to poor transformation of food, or nourishment is cut off by stagnation.

Remedy Protect the Fetus and Aid Life powder

Ingredients   *ren shen, bai zhu, fu ling, zhi gan cao, shan yao, bai bian dou, lian zi, yi yi ren, bai dou kou, huo xiang, ze xie, mai ya, jie geng, chen pi, shan zha, huang lian,* and *qian shi*

Cause   Qi and blood deficiencies. A weakness of the reproductive system due to general deficiencies of Qi and blood

Remedy Powder that Gives the Stability of Mount Tai

Ingredients ren shen, huang qi, xu duan, huang qin, chuan xiong, shu di huang, bai shao, bai zhu, zhi gan cao, sha ren, and glutinous rice

Cause restless fetus with vaginal bleeding. Liver blood deficiency causes the blood to become disordered.

Remedy Enhanced Four Substances

Ingredients shu di huang, bai shao, dang gui, chuan xiong, ai ye, and e jiao

Cause damage to the *chong* and *ren*. This is injury or trauma to the reproductive system. The *chong* and *ren* are the acupuncture channels that generally nourish the reproductive organs.

Remedy normal herbs for injury are contraindicated

Injury, Trauma, and Pain

Experiences passed on from generation to generation have given Chinese doctors a unique understanding of injury and the healing process. Over thousands of years, monks and soldiers developed methods to aid recovery from injury sustained during their respective martial arts training and combat. Their practice is called *Dit Da Yao* (hit medicine). Here are a few of their secrets.

Disease Condition   Injuries progress through three stages. The first stage lasts up to two days after the injury, the second stage a few weeks. Injuries older than two weeks are considered third stage or old injuries. Treatment must be appropriate for each stage.

At first, treatment must stop bleeding, clear debris, cool heat (reduce inflammation), vitalize blood (relieve pain), and protect against stagnation by promoting the flow of energy and fluids to the injured area. First-stage treatment can employ electro-acupuncture near the site of the injury as well as internal and topical herbs. At all stages of injury, the Chinese practitioner uses acupuncture, herbs, and massage instead of ice as a means of reducing swelling. When the injury looks red or feels warm to the touch, heat is never applied, nor is ice. Herbs are used to clear the heat. Ice restricts flow at a time when flow is required to clear debris. TCM practitioners believe that using ice could result in poorly healed tissue with pain persisting into the second and third stages. Soaking is also discouraged whenever swelling is present, as it will worsen the swelling.

Herbal and Non-Herbal Treatments

Stage One of Injury   Internal herbal medicines for first-stage injuries are *Tieh Ta Wan, Jin Gu Die Shang Wan, Chin Koo Tieh Shang Wan,* and *Yunnan Baiyao* capsules.

Stage Two of Injury   In the second stage, several days after the trauma, practitioners continue to clear heat, reduce swelling, break remaining stagnations, promote flow, and begin to strengthen the Qi of the tissue. Gentle acupuncture will promote flow, relieve pressure, and loosen stagnations. Herbs that promote the flow of water and herbs to disperse Qi (energy) at the surface will be used topically to reduce any remaining swelling. Massage, which may have been too painful in the first stage, will be used in the second stage to aid the movement of energy and fluids. Some products for second-stage injury are Dr. Shin's Liniment made by Spring Wind Herbs, and Seven Forest's San Qi 17 pills.

Stage Three of Injury   In the third stage, when the injury is severe or has been improperly treated, the site will be weak due to poor flow-through and insufficient nourishment. At this stage, the area must be strengthened to facilitate better flow. Pain is from cold rather than heat, as the inflammation was resolved by this stage. The task is to warm the channels. Here moxibustion (heat treatment, see Chapter 1, "Methods of Chinese Medicine") is at least as valuable as acupuncture. Massage and strengthening herbs like *dang gui,* drynaria, and eucommia are used internally and externally. Sometimes herbs used for arthritis (wind damp herbs), such as *du huo* (cow parsnip root) or *qin jiao (gentian)*, are also employed.

Notes   Most of the products used for injury are contraindicated for pregnancy.

Topical herbs: Some of the best poultices are made in the United

States by Spring Wind Herbs. Called soft plasters, these trauma ointments are applied to an injury, covered, and taped in place for several days. Formulas are available for each stage and to accomplish various medical tasks, such as reducing swelling or inflammation.

Insomnia, Anxiety, and Restlessness

Disease Condition   Short-term problems of insomnia are caused by noise, excitement, schedules, medicines, caffeine, alcohol, and other stimulations of modern life. However, 10 percent of us suffer from chronic, long-term sleep disorders, which are a more elusive problem for modern medicine. Despite having developed many drugs that put people to sleep, chronic disorders remain a mystery to Western medicine. Sleeplessness is not as mysterious to Chinese medicine, having refined its understanding of this symptom. Insomnia is not a disease but is rather the symptom of disharmony. Some patterns causing symptoms of insomnia and their treatments are as follows:

Disturbed Shen   The spirit resides in the heart and is called the *shen*. During times of stress, constraint occurs in the chest causing heat to gather near the heart, disturbing the *shen* and making one feel restless, sleepless, ill tempered, or just out of sorts. Besides insomnia, this condition can also cause headache, dizziness, heart palpitations, and poor concentration. Good remedies are Dr. Shen's Good Sleep and Worry-Free pills to nourish and clear heat from the heart, or An Mien Pian (Peaceful Sleep pill). Versions are made by China National Native Produce and Animal-by-Products in Hebei, China, Plum Flower, Herbal Times, and others.

Heart Blood Deficiency   Blood deficiencies do not always show up on blood tests and are often diagnosed by their symptoms, which include weak pulse, pale tongue, pale lips, dry skin, fatigue, and insomnia. Poor blood fails to properly nourish the heart (mind), causing insomnia. Those with this type of insomnia have difficulty falling asleep, may be especially tired in the afternoons or after eating, and could have a digestive complaint as well. Commonly used medicines include *gui pi wan* and *suan zao ren wan*. Both of these are available wherever Chinese herbs are sold.

Deficiency Heat Common during menopause, this kind of insomnia is caused by heat. However, this heat is an experience that comes from a deficiency of yin (cool) rather than a true excess of heat (fever). The body remains at about 98.6 degrees. Here, the yin cooling system is insufficient to offset the body's normal metabolic heat. Hot flashes or waking at night feeling warm are warnings of weakened yin. The mind alerts you to this condition by momentarily allowing you to experience your body's hot, 98.6-degree temperature. To remedy this type of insomnia, combine Good Sleep pills with *zhi bai di huang wan* or Er Xiang Wan (Two Immortals pill).

Disharmony Between Heart and Kidneys Insomnia caused by weak kidneys that affect the heart and lead to disturbed *shen* (see Chapter 3, "Understanding Theories of Chinese Medicine," The Twelve Organs) can be accompanied by symptoms of vivid dreams or nightmares, heart palpitations, or anxiety. It can also be accompanied by heat in the kidneys that causes heightened, or difficult to satisfy, sexual desire. Use Tian Wang Bu Xin Dan pills to treat this condition. This classical formula is also known as Emperor's Teapills. Many brands are available.

Irritable Bowel Syndrome (IBS)

IBS is a catch-all diagnosis for intestinal complaints not understood by your doctor. When the diagnosis is IBS, it may mean your doctor does not know what is causing your problems. It means that tests such as colonoscopies and X-rays have revealed no other disease.

In contrast, Chinese medicine has more experience in understanding and treating these ailments. Practitioners do not consider IBS symptoms, such as diarrhea, constipation, cramps, and bloating, to be mysterious. All pertain to the free flow of energy and fluids (Qi and blood), or the timing and balance of the digestive organs (yin and yang). These patterns, a puzzle to many in the Western world, are well documented in the annals of Chinese medicine: Spleen Qi Deficiency, Spleen Yang Deficiency, Damp Heat in the Large Intestine, Liver Qi Stagnation, Liver Invades Spleen, and Liver Invades Stomach.

Since these differing patterns are all called IBS by modern medicine, the diagnosis provides little help to a practitioner of Chinese medicine. Rather, The Four Examinations are used. (See Chapter 3, "Understanding Theories of Chinese Medicine)."

Herbal Treatments There are few credible herbal remedies to treat IBS. You can find great medicines for Spleen Deficiency, Liver Invades Stomach, and for specific complaints like constipation or diarrhea (see the Digestive Problems section of this chapter), but no retail formula can treat all the unique patterns that could be included in a diagnosis of IBS.

Calm Colon, a formula shown to be effective for IBS in a controlled study done at Samra University in Southern California, was intensely marketed several years ago It was a huge formulation, designed to cover any possible source of IBS. The company that originally made the product is out of business, but many people still look for it. Though Dr. Shen's practice has no direct experience using it, a Dr. Shen's brand version is now being manufactured to satisfy requests for the formula. The ingredients are: white peony root, fragrant angelica root, white atractylodes root, hare's ear root, plantain seed, tangerine peel, codonopsis root, siler root, Hoelin mushroom, polyporus mushroom, phelodendron bark, goldenthread root, magnolia bark, patchouli plant, costus root, ginger root, Chinese ash bark, schisandra berry, Job's tears seed, capillary artimesia leaves, and Chinese licorice root.

Non-Herbal Treatments Acupuncture, which affects the Qi directly, quickly helps many IBS complaints. Perhaps this is because these patterns tend to be Qi-related rather than organic. Were they organic, they would have a medical definition and not be called IBS. Since IBS can mean many different things, it is hard to predict exactly how an acupuncturist will treat it. You can expect some points to be selected on the abdomen and along the stomach and spleen channels that lie on either side of the shins.

Lice

Herbal Treatment Throw away your pesticides and forget about tea tree oil and other herbs that rarely work. A combination of two

Chinese herbs—*bai bu* and *ku shen*—used according to the directions provided, stops itching and kills lice and their nits (eggs) overnight—guaranteed. These herbs should be boiled and used fresh each time. If they are allowed to stay in the fridge, they will loose their potency. Prepared extracts, such as tinctures, are also likely to be ineffectual. We sell this mixture under the name of No More Lice Herbal Soak. However, you can save money by doing this yourself. The herbs are cheap, easy to find, and absolutely nontoxic to humans.

Ingredients

Kills lice stemona root, *bai bu*, 80 percent

Stops itch sophora root, *ku shen*, 20 percent

Directions Shortly before bedtime, boil two ounces of chopped whole dried herbs in five cups of water for thirty minutes. The cooking pot can be ceramic, glass, or stainless steel. Never use aluminum or iron pots to cook medicinal herbs. Stir occasionally, and watch the pot to prevent boiling over. Strain, and allow liquid to cool. After the medicine has cooled to body temperature, apply it generously to the hair and scalp immediately. Do not allow the liquid to sit for hours before use. Next, cover hair with shower cap or towel. Finally, go to sleep. The herbs will ease any itch. After soaking overnight, shampoo and comb out dead nits with a fine-tooth comb. Repeat when necessary. Though this product most often works on the first application, a second application in one week can often help prevent recurrence.

Be sure to also take all other precautions, such as removing and laundering clothes and bedding.

Menopause and Hot Flashes

Disease Condition To understand menopause, forget about hormones and survey your body in terms of yin and yang (see Chapter 3, "Understanding Theories of Chinese Medicine"). Menopause is yin deficiency.

Activity, movement, and metabolism are called yang. Yang metabolic activity generates friction and heat inside the body. Bodies require circulating fluids, known as the yin, to cool and insulate us from this heat. The kidney yin has been described as a mist that cools the heart, liver, lungs, stomach, and intestines. When this yin is deficient, you'll feel the heat or the effects of the heat: dry, constipated, and agitated. You may also feel exhausted: wired and tired. Your sex drive will probably be diminished, though there are cases where the opposite is true. The syndrome of feeling hot because your cooling system is weak has many names: Yin Deficiency Fire, Vacuity Fire, Deficiency Heat, Weak Heat, False Fire, and other similar terms.

Deficiency fire can be distinguished from excess fire by the lack of an elevated body temperature, a red tongue tip versus a red tongue body, and a weak pulse rather than a bold one. Generally, yin deficiency heat is long-term, whereas excess heat comes from a sudden illness, like a flu or malarial disorder.

In truth, menopause is never simply yin-deficient heat. After approximately fifty years of life, a person arrives at menopause with a complex set of deficiencies and discomforts. Hot flashes, night sweats, low libido, dryness, insomnia, fatigue, moodiness, neck and shoulder tension, depression, anxiety, and high blood pressure are among the most common. Some of these are caused by diminished yang, Qi, and blood, as well as by deficient yin. It may be helpful to see menopause as an individual pattern in which the yin is more deficient than the yang.

These patterns are always longstanding and are far easier to prevent than to treat. Remember the adage about waiting until you are thirsty before digging the well. Cultivate and preserve yin with rest and harmony when you are forty. It will pay off when you are fifty.

Non-Herbal Treatments Acupuncture is useful for menopause because it can clear heat. Needles placed in the fleshy part of the hand, between the thumb and forefinger (*he gu*), cool and relieve pain in the upper body. Pricking the tip of the third finger and drawing out a few drops of blood cools fever and can relieve insomnia. Prick all the fingers to chill out manic behavior, usually within minutes.

Herbal Treatment Chinese herbs contain no hormones, yet they relieve menopausal problems. Seen from the perspective of practioners of Chinese medicine, these herbs provide relief by correcting imbalances of the yin, yang, Qi, and blood. Such imbalances are the cause of hormonal imbalances and are the root of most menopausal complaints. Hormones may relieve symptoms, but they cannot harmonize yin and yang, and hormones can cause cancer. When Chinese herbs and acupuncture work for you, they are far better medicine than hormones.

Black cohosh (*sheng ma*) is a Chinese herb found in many Western herbal products used for menopause. Though it reduces hot flashes effectively, it is badly misused for this purpose. Black cohosh should be used only for short periods of time to reduce excess heat from fevers. Long-term use of this herb is not recommended.

The heat experienced from hot flashes is long-term and caused by a weak cooling system. It is different from the heat of fevers requiring black cohosh. There are many better herbs than black cohosh (*sheng ma*) for deficiency heat. The most notable is Anemarrhena (*zhi mu*), which reduces hot flashes and builds the yin of the body at the same time. For menopause, Anemarrhena is more therapeutic and safer than black cohosh.

The following herbal supplements are used for menopause and are believed to supplement and harmonize yin and yang and to clear deficiency heat. They are quite different from one another in composition and approach, but are absolutely safe, readily available, and all well worth testing out before resorting to hormone therapy.

Er Xiang Wan (Two Immortals pill, see chapter 5, "Famous Herbal Medicines"), Plum Flower, and Dr. Shen's. Dr. Shen's version contains a small amount of oyster shell.

- Da Bu Yin Wan (Great Yin Tonifying pill). Uses turtle shell to tonify the yin. Many brands available.
- *Zhi bai di huang wan* (Rehmannia Eight pill, see Chapter 5, "Famous Herbal Medicines"). Many brands available.
- *He che da zao wan* (Placenta Restorative pills). May contain human placenta. Lanzhou and Guangzhou versions available.
- *Geng nian an wan* (Menopause Comfort pill). Uses pearl (*zhen zhu mu*) and wheat berries (*fu xiao mai*) to clear heat and stop sweating. Bio Essence brand.
- *Zuo Gui Wan* (Left Return pills). Classical formula for yin deficiency. Kwangchow, Herbal Times, Plum Flower, and Bio Essence brands.

Nausea, Vomiting, Gastric Reflux, and Morning Sickness

Disease Condition   Digestive Qi obviously moves downward. We feel nauseous when some of our digestive Qi is moving upward instead of downward. This phenomena is called rebellious stomach Qi, and it causes nausea and vomiting. Other kinds of rebellious Qi cause sneezing, coughing, and hiccups. Stomach Qi rebels for many reasons: food stagnation, weak digestive Qi, attacks from the liver, obstruction in the intestines, and pressure from a developing fetus, to name a few. Symptoms of indigestion, gastric reflux disease, stomach flu, hangover, and morning sickness are all related to rebellious stomach Qi.

Non-Herbal Treatments   Acupuncture has been shown to relieve nausea and vomiting resulting from chemotherapy and morning sickness. At least one insurance company has approved acupuncture for these conditions. Dr. Shen's practice always treats morning sickness using acupuncture, though usually favors herbal treatment for those undergoing chemotherapy.

Chinese herbal medicine is far ahead of Western medicine in the treatment of all the conditions mentioned above. Proof of this can easily be found in the humble and ubiquitous Stomach Curing pill, which requires no diagnosis to use or prescription to obtain.

Stomach Curing pills (also known as Po Chai pills) are a fixture in most medicine cabinets in China and are considered a must for travelers. Use them for acute nausea from stomach flu, indigestion, hangover, or motion sickness. Do not use them for acid regurgitation, gastric reflux disease, or for chronic complaints. They work quickly and reliably, usually within fifteen minutes. Stomach Curing pills are convincing evidence of how effective herbs can be. Several brands are available, including Dr. Shen's, Plum Flower, and Herbal Times. Ingredients and their functions are listed below to show their complexity.

Stomach Curing pills evolved from *bao he wan* (Preserve Harmony pill) which first appeared in *The Teachings of Zhu*, by Zhu Zheng Heng, 1481.

Ingredients of Stomach Curing pills

- Costus root (*mu xiang, Saussureae radix*): moves the Qi, dissipates stagnant intestinal Qi, and alleviates pain.
- Angelica root (*bai zhi, Angelica dahurica*): expels wind, releases surface, alleviates pain, reduces swelling, expels dampness, and alleviates discharge.
- Medicated leaven (*shen qu, Massa fermentata*): dissolves food, transforms accumulations, and aids digestion.
- Mint leaf (*bo he, Mentha folium*): frees constrained Qi, clears the head and eyes, and disperses wind heat.
- Citrus peel (*chen pi, Citri rubrum exocarpum*): moves the Qi, strengthens spleen, dries dampness, directs the Qi downward, and prevents stagnation.
- Chrysanthemum (*ju hua, Chrysanthemomi flos*): disperses wind, clears heat from the eyes, and pacifies the liver.
- Ornamental orchid (*tian ma, Gastrodia rhiz*): pacifies the liver, extinguishes wind, alleviates pain, and disperses painful obstruction.
- Hoelin mushroom (*fu ling, Poria cocos*): quiets the heart, calms the spirit, harmonizes the middle, and strengthens stomach/spleen.
- Job's tears (*yi yi ren, coix lachryma jobi*): leaches dampness, strengthens stomach/spleen, clears damp heat, and reduces diarrhea.
- Magnolia bark (*hou po, Magnolia cortex*): moves the Qi, transforms dampness, resolves stagnation, and directs rebellious Qi downward.
- Patchouli (*huo xiang, Agastach pogostemi*): transforms dampness, releases the exterior, harmonizes the center, and expels dampness.
- White Atractylodes (*bai zhu, Atractylodes radix*): benefits the Qi, stabilizes the exterior, strengthens the spleen, and dries dampness.
- Rice sprout (*gu ya, Oryzae germinantus*): dissolves food stagnation and strengthens stomach.
- Kudzu root (*ge gen, Pueraria radix*): clears heat, releases muscles of upper body, and nourishes fluids.

Besides Stomach Curing pills, there are many other medicines for nausea, vomiting, and other causes of rebellious stomach Qi. Here are some of the more well-known and easy to find formulations:

Herbal Formulas for Nausea

Xiang sha yang wei wan (aucklandia, Amomum Nourish Stomach pill): classic formula and an excellent general digestive tonic. Minshan, Herbal Times, Tanglong, Lanzhou, and other brands.

Gan Lu Qing Re Pian (Sweet Dew Clear Heat tablet): good and fast for nausea and vomiting from food poisoning. Sing-Kyn Drug House, Guangzhou, China.

Fu zi li zhong wan (Aconitum Compound pills): used for weak digestive Qi. Lanzhou, Tanglong, United, and other versions.

Single Herbs for Nausea Ginger (*sheng jiang*), pinellia (*ban xia*), perilla leaf (*su ye*), patchouli (*huo xiang*), citrus peel (*chen pi*), amomi seed (*sha ren*), and cardamom (*bai dou kou*).

Pain

Disease Condition Where there's pain, there's no flow. The message of pain is always the same, no matter what condition it may be associated with. Pain means that normal flow of Qi or blood is inhibited, that something is stuck. When flow is interrupted, pain alerts you. Where you think nerve, practitioners of Chinese medicine notice the flow associated with that nerve. When the flow is like a river, full and flowing, everything thrives. When it's not flowing, you're hurting.

It doesn't take a genius to understand or fix this problem, nor does it require endless drugs. To relieve pain, we discern why the river isn't flowing properly. Then we treat it. Our tools are acupuncture, moxibustion, massage, herbs, and movement. Like everything else in Chinese medicine, techniques vary according to individual circumstances. The diagnosis will come from observing the river.

Pain may be caused by:

Obstruction Like a tree fallen in the river, an injury, swelling, or accumulation can block or divert the flow.

Constraint A river may narrow and constrain the flow of water; so, also, does tension, which constricts the channels and constrains the flow of Qi and blood.

Deficiency As the river dries, it cannot flow, and stagnant pools collect. Likewise, empty Qi and blood become stagnant Qi and blood.

Non-Herbal Treatments Acupuncture invigorates the Qi, moves the blood, and thus relieves pain, making it central for treatment plans aimed at pain relief. Vigorous Asian massage techniques like Shiatsu and Tui Na (see Chapter 1, "Methods of Chinese Medicine") are also aimed at moving Qi and blood. They are more effective at alleviating pain than simple muscle massage.

Herbal Treatment Most of the herbs used to relieve pain fall into two categories: Herbs that Move Blood and Herbs that Move Qi. Pain from blood stagnation is fixed in one spot and usually intense, whereas pain from Qi stagnation is more likely to move and is usually (but not always) less intense. For abdominal pain due to poor flow of food, Herbs that Relieve Food Stagnation are also used (see Chapter 7, "Herbs and Their Categories").

The strongest herb for relieving pain is the resin of *ying su hua (Papaveris somniferi)*. We know it as opium. The second most potent is the legal herb *yan hu suo (Corydalis rhizome)*, said to have less than half the power of codeine. Stronger effects are achieved by combining herbs into formulas. Using formulas rather than single herbs also permits adding herbs that modify the unwanted side effects of some herbs. Most blood vitalizing herbs, for example, are extremely bitter and can cause nausea or are contraindicated for pregnancy. Formulas can also target specific parts of the body or specific syndromes.

The following general pain medicines will relieve pain better than any single herb (except opium). However, herbs taken internally will not often equal the blessedly fast and reliable action of three ibuprofen tablets.

General Pain Medicines

Yan hu suo wan Formulas containing *yan hu suo* can be used for any kind of pain but are most effective for toothache and headache. All versions are contraindicated during pregnancy. Variations are available from many manufacturers. The Sing Kyn, Xing Qun, and Yukiang versions contain berberine, an alkaloid extracted from this herb. These versions are illegal in California.

Qi Ye Lian analgesic pills   Schefflera Root Relieve Pain tablets are 100 percent *qi ye lian (Schefflera arboricola)*. This herb is of recent discovery, so there is little history of its use. Nevertheless, it is said to relieve pain safely, without toxicity. Versions from Heping Pharmaceutical and Plum Flower are available.

China tung shueh pills   China's Painful Blood pills are used for pain from poor circulation in the joints or lumbar region of the spine. This medicine is popular in China for treatment of arthritis or pain from old injuries. Use the Plum Flower version. Be careful to avoid Cow's Head brand, manufactured in Taiwan. It has been found to contain diazepam (Valium), chlormezanone (tranquilizers), and clorzoxazone (a muscle relaxant). The version made by Kwangchow Pharmaceutical in Guangzhou has also been found to contain chemicals and excess heavy metals.

Also avoid *jin bu huan* anodyne tablets made by Pai Se Pharmaceutical in Guangxi. These are actually the alkaloid tetrahydropalmatini sulphate extracted from the herb *jin bu huan*. Though they do relieve pain, they are narcotic and hypnotic. Overdoses have required emergency room visits. Banned by the FDA, it should be regarded as an unapproved drug rather than as an herb.

Prostate Conditions

Traditional Chinese Medicine views the prostate gland as part of the kidney organ system, combining the urinary, reproductive, nervous, and skeletal systems (see The Twelve Organs in Chapter 3, "Understanding Theories of Chinese Medicine"). From a modern point of view, prostate complaints fall into three main types: enlarged prostate, prostatitis (painful prostate), and prostate cancer. Practioners of Traditional Chinese Medicine view it differently.

Disease Conditions and Their Herbal Treatments

Types of Prostate Conditions

1. Excess Type: Acute Prostatitis. Pain, burning urination, dark urine, pus, blood, or strong odor are characteristic of the excess type. The pulse may be rapid. The tongue may be red, or the tongue coating may be yellow. Acute prostatitis is caused by pathogenic bacteria, virus, or other invasive organisms or toxins.

Pain can be diminished using acupuncture or electro-acupuncture near the site of the pain or discomfort. Needles may also be placed on the insides of the legs or ankles. Heat treatment (moxibustion) is forbidden, because this is an inflamed condition. Herbs that clear heat and those that clean toxins, normally used for infection and inflammation, are used for this condition.

Ba Zheng Wan (Eight Righteous pills) is the most traditional formula for symptoms of prostatitis, but not always the most reliable. If your symptoms remain after a few days, you may want to try a course of antibiotics. If you've already tried antibiotics and they have not been successful, you may actually have the deficiency type of prostatitis.

2. Deficiency type prostatitis presents with chronic discomfort, pressure, distention, and frequent or dribbling urination. The urine is neither dark nor odorous; rather, it is pale and plentiful. This condition is usually diagnosed as benign prostate hypertrophy (BPH). It is caused by kidney or spleen yang deficiency. Men with deficiency types might also have a slow or weak pulse, a pale tongue, a thick tongue coating, weak digestion, lower back weakness, or low sexual desire.

These two herbal medicines for deficiency type prostrate problems are best taken in combination:

Kai Kit Prostate Gland pill Different versions are made by Hanyang Pharmaceutical Works, Hanyang; Peoples Pharmaceutical Factory, Wuzhou; and Herbal Times, Bio Essence, Plum Flower, and others.

Golden Book pill Also used to treat other forms of kidney deficiency. Almost every manufacturer makes a version of this formula (see Chapter 5, "Famous Herbal Medicines").

3. Prostate Cancer Type: There has been great interest in a Chinese formula called PC-SPES (PC is short for prostate cancer, and Spes is the Roman goddess of hope). Studies showed that it dramatically lowers prostate specific antigen (PSA) levels in patients with advanced prostate cancer. Rising PSA levels in the blood are thought to indicate the presence and expansion of prostate cancer. Interestingly, these reports appeared in the *New England Journal of Medicine*, not as a breakthrough for herbal medicine, but rather as a caution to doctors that herbs could powerfully affect hormones and were therefore an unregulated hazard.

Proponents of the drug claimed that it achieves its effect because of its immune enhancing and cancer fighting properties. However, certain problems about this therapy have since come to light. First, it achieves its PSA lowering effect by affecting hormones, rather than through any anti-cancer or immune enhancing effect. Second, it turns out not to be an herbal drug. In 2002, the FDA recalled the product when it discovered that it contained one or more pharmaceutical agents.

Real treatment of prostate cancer with Chinese herbs is according to the principle of *fu zheng gu ben*. *Fu zheng* means strengthening what is correct. *Gu ben* means regeneration and repair (see the Cancer section of this chapter).

Sexual Problems

Erectile disfunction and premature ejaculation are examples of low sexual function. These problems can have emotional or biological roots. When biology is the root cause, low sexual function is usually caused by kidney yang deficiency, but it may also be caused by yin or *jing* deficiency. This is true for both men and women.

As the kidneys are said to be the repository of Qi, they are often named in deficiency conditions. Having a kidney deficiency is like having low batteries or a dwindling bank account. Such vacuities are caused by spending more energy than can be replenished. When this occurs, reserves are tapped and eventually depleted. Excessive spending of energy on work, thought, physical trauma, sexual activity, or emotional turbulence will eventually cause this depletion. Digestive problems will speed its occurrence. Poor or insufficient sleep, failure to rejuvenate through rest or vacation, and congenital deficiencies can also play a part.

Kidney yang deficiency can also result in low sperm count, poor sperm motility, bed-wetting, feeling cold at the core, or exhaustion following ejaculation. It is sometimes accompanied by a sense of fatigue that is largely unrelieved by sleep, frequent urination, or weakness in the lower back or lower body. Kidney *jing* deficiency is marked by premature graying or aging.

Herbal Treatments Remedies for sexual problems caused by kidney yang and *jing* deficiency include:

Man's Treasure formulas (nan bao) Many versions of this formula are available in Chinese herb stores. Some formulas are huge, containing over thirty herbs. Some contain the genitalia of dogs, deer, or seals. Some contain seahorse or pipefish. Dr. Shen's, Seven Forest, Health Concerns, Planetary Herbs, Evergreen Herbs, and other American manufacturers make animal-free versions.

Kidney yin deficiency stems from aging, overwork, loss of fluids, or excessive sexual activity. Patients often feel warm, wired, and tired. Kidney yin deficiency can also cause impotence in men or women, and reduced ejaculate in men or vaginal dryness in women. The formulas *liu we di huang* and *zhi bai di huang* are used for kidney yin deficiencies. For low libido with heat signs associated with menopause or aging, take Two Immortals pills (see Chapter 5, "Famous Herbal Medicines"). Men may also take this pill.

Thyroid Problems

Disease Conditions Thyroid diseases are the symptoms of deeper imbalances called kidney deficiencies. The kidneys are said to be the repository of Qi (energy) and supply this energy to various organs and glands (see The Twelve Organs in Chapter 3, "Understanding

Theories of Chinese Medicine"). When the thyroid gland is under-supplied, it malfunctions, producing diverse patterns of hormonal se-cretions and thus a wide variety of symptoms.

Hyperthyroid, Graves' disease, and some thyroid cancers are caused primarily by an undersupply of yin. Yin fluids cool the heat produced by your body's metabolism (activity). The result of yin deficiency is often de-ficiency heat. Though it cannot be measured on a thermometer, this kind of heat can agitate your body, triggering glandular activity and a constel-lation of symptoms. Hot flashes, tidal fevers, insomnia, restlessness, and hyperthyroid can occur because the yin is insufficient to cool the yang.

Hypothyroid, Hashimoto's complex, and some goiters are diagnosed when the kidney yang is deficient. Yang refers to your body's metabo-lism, movement, activity, and fire. When yang is low, lethargy and cold result, circulation is poor, and glands tend to be underproductive.

Herbal Treatment   Herbs and acupuncture can both be useful in restoring yin/yang harmony to the body. For those who do not have access to professional help, the following herbal formulas and herbal products have been selected because they are safe for general use.

Herbal Formula for Hyperthyroid
gui ban: turtle shell, seven grams
hai zao: seaweed, seven grams
kun bu: alga, seven grams
zhi mu: anamarenna root, seven grams
zhi zi: gardenia seed, seven grams
xuan shen: scrophularia, seven grams
da zao: Chinese dates, seven grams
mu li: oyster shell, seven grams
Amounts are given for herb granules. Mix herbs together. Take three grams two or three times a day

Products
Zuo Gui pills (Left Return pill): many sources available
Zhi Bai Di Huang Wan: (see Chapter 5, "Famous Herbal Medicines")
Da Bu Yin Wan (Great Yin Tonifying pill): many versions available

Herbal Formula for Hypothyroid

hai zao: seaweed or *kun bu*: algae, seven grams

shu di huang: cooked rehmannia root, seven grams

shan zhu yu: cornus fruit, seven grams

shan yao: yam root, seven grams

fu zi: prepared aconite root, five grams

rou gui: cinnamon bark, five grams

ze xie: water plantain rhizome, seven grams

fu ling: *Poria cocos*, seven grams

mu dan pi: tree peony bark, seven grams

Doses are given for herb granules. Mix herbs together. Take three grams two or three times a day.

Herbal Formula for Benign Tumors of the Thyroid

hai zao: seaweed, seven grams

kun bu: algae, seven grams

hai dai: laminaria, seven grams

zhi bei mu: fritillaria thunbergi bulb, seven grams

ban xia: pinellia tuber, seven grams

jie geng: balloon flower root, seven grams

chuan xiong: liguisticum, seven grams

qing pi: unripe citus peel, seven grams

chen pi: citrus peel, five grams

lian qiao: forsythia fruit, seven grams

gan cao: licorice root, three grams

Doses given for herb granules. Mix herbs together. Take three grams two or three times a day

Vaginal Yeast Infections

Disease Condition   In the book *Fire in the Valley: The Traditional Chinese Medical Diagnosis and Treatment of Vaginal Diseases*, author Bob Flaws notes that diagnosis for most vaginal yeast infections (candidiasis) is damp heat in the lower burner. The yeast organism is a fungus, and, like all fungi, craves a damp environment. You'll find mushrooms (fungi) after the rain in a damp forest, but you'll never find one in the desert. In your body, excessive water will cause fungal and other pathogens to flourish. We call this condition internal dampness. Curing yeast infections requires drying dampness more than it requires killing fungi. Experience shows that these conditions are stubborn and hard to treat; hence the expression "dampness is difficult."

The common causes of excessive damp include poor digestion that allows excess moisture to remain in the body; excessive consumption of cold foods, raw foods, and dairy products, which produce damp internal conditions; and insufficient fire (internal cold). Without enough metabolic fire to steam off water, damp can accumulate.

Acupuncture may be helpful in relieving some of the itching and pain that can accompany this condition, but it is not usually a cure. Herbal medicine may be more helpful.

Herbal Treatment Yeast infections may exist with either excess or deficient conditions. The principal sign of vaginal yeast infections is called leukorrhea (yellow discharge). This indicates an excess condition. However, many women with yeast infections have white vaginal discharge, clear discharge, or no discharge at all. These distinctions can help distinguish excess from deficiency, and dampness from heat. Red, brown, or yellow discharge indicates heat, whereas white or clear discharge shows more dampness. No discharge hints at deficiency as one of the root causes. Other distinctions are made using the Four Examinations (see Chapter 1, "Methods of Chinese Medicine"). This rounds out the diagnosis and suggests the best course of treatment. Though it may take an herbologist to prepare an individual prescription, the following medicines are safe for everyone, and will do no harm if improperly prescribed:

Yudai wan Use for excess conditions, such as invasion of heat toxins (trichomonas or candida albicans). Contains 47 percent *chun pi* (alianthus), an astringent herb known for its effectiveness against trichomonas. Minshan, Lanzhou Foci, Tanglong, and Bio Essence brands.

Chien chin chih tai wan Use for damp heat in the lower burner caused by deficiency and marked by clear, white, cloudy, or curd-like discharge. Tianjin and Plum Flower brands.

Lung tan xie gan wan Use to clear damp heat from the liver or gallbladder channel. The liver channel passes through the genitals, and the connecting gallbladder channel passes through the ears. That's why this formula, oddly, treats both genital problems and ear problems. It is not used for liver or gallbladder organ problems. It is used for earaches and for genital herpes as well as for all kinds of vaginal infections. Minshan, Kwangchow Herbal Times, Plum Flower, and Tanglong brands.

To make your own formula, use equal parts of the following herbs:

Phellodendron amurense	*huang bai*	amur cork tree	clears heat, dries damp
Gentiana scabrae	*long dan cao*	gentian root	clears heat, dries damp
Coix lachryma jobi	*yi yi ren*	Job's tears	drains damp
Glycyrrhiza uralensis	*gan cao*	licorice root	tonifies Qi

For yellow or brown vaginal discharge add:

Coptis chinensis	*huang lian*	golden thread	clears heat, dries damp
Taraxaci mongolici	*pu gong yin*	dandelion	clears heat, cleans toxins

To treat vaginal itching add:

Sophora flavescens	*ku shen*	bitter root	clears heat, dries damp

For white or clear vaginal discharge add:

Atractylodes alba	*bai zhu*	Atractylodes root	tonifies Qi
Poria cocos	*fu ling*	Hoelen fungus	drains damp
Codonopsis pilosula	*dang shen*	codonopsis root	tonifies Qi

For vaginal dryness or itching with no discharge add:

Paeonia lactiflora	*bai shao*	white peony root	tonifies blood
Angelica sinenses	*dang gui*	tang kwei	tonifies blood

Warts

Warts (*Verruca vulgaris*) are called *wian ri chuang* (thousand day sores). According to Western medicine, they are a form of viral vegetation. According to Chinese medicine, warts are caused by lingering pathogenic wind in the skin that is in turn caused by liver blood deficiency.

Topical treatments for common warts, flat warts, filliform warts, and plantar warts:

1. Burn direct with moxa (see Chapter 1, "Methods of Chinese Medicine").

2. Wash and rub with a decoction of thirty grams of *mu zei* (*Herba equestri*) and thirty grams of *xiang fu* (*Rhizoma cyperi*). Boil thirty minutes in 1,500 mililiters (about 1.5 quarts) of water. Apply two times per day for thirty minutes each time.

3. Smash a kernel of *ya dan zi* (*Fructus bruceae*) to expose the oily interior. Protect the surrounding skin with petroleum jelly, then apply the oil to the wart once every other day. Be careful! This oil is extremely caustic. Rub the wart once a day with chicken gizzard (*endothelium corni*), after it has been soaked in water.

Internal herbs for warts You must not use internal herbs for warts during pregnancy. When not pregnant, use equal parts of:

Magnetitum	*ci shi*	loadstone	settles the spirit
Margaritifera zhen	*zhu mu*	mother of pearl	settles the spirit
Ostrera concha	*mu li*	oyster shell	settles the spirit
Carthami flos	*hong ua*	safflower	vitalizes blood
Persica semen	*tao ren*	peach kernel	vitalizes blood
Squama manitis	*sang piao xiao*	mantis egg case	astringent
Gleditsia sinensis	*zao jiao*	honeylocust fruit	relieves coughing, wheezing
Lonicera japonica	*jin yin hua*	honeysuckle	clears heat, cleans toxins
Phellodendron amurense	*huang bai*	amur cork tree bark	clears heat, dries damp

Internal formula for liver blood deficiency:

Paeonia lactiflora	*bai shao*	white peony root	tonifies blood
Angelica sinenses	*dang gui*	tang kwei	tonifies blood
Lycium chinense	*gou qi zi*	go ji berry	tonifies blood
Atractylodes alba	*bai zhu*	Atractylodes root	tonifies Qi

Weight Gain, Weight Loss, and Diets

The Chinese spend a lot of time preparing, talking about, and eating food, yet overweight people are rare in China. Westerners also spend a lot of time preparing, talking about, and eating food—but they suffer from widespread obesity. Perhaps there's a lesson here about how to eat well and be slim. From the point of view of Chinese medicine and observations of Asian culture, being slim has a lot to do with how you eat. Learning and adopting good eating habits, including those of moderation and temperance, is a sure and permanent cure for obesity. Changing eating habits, however, is much harder than following a diet. The following are Dr. Shen's diet recomendations for those who choose to make a change:

Enjoy food   Prepare your own food, pay attention to the taste and quality of food you eat, and spend more time eating. You will be satisfied by less food.

Eat regularly   Your body adjusts to regular events. Timing is important for good digestion, providing more energy from less food.

Enjoy hunger   Don't panic when hunger arrives. You're not really starving. Hunger is the feeling of loosing weight, so when you are fat, hunger is good for you.

Eat Chinese   People in China rarely eat the huge portions of deep-fried delights you typically find in American Chinese restaurants. They eat mainly rice, noodles, vegetables, and a little meat or seafood. Eat only this and you will not gain weight.

Enrich your life   There are other pleasures in life besides food. Add something pleasurable to your life. Learn something, do something different, start something, go somewhere. Challenge yourself.

Be vigilant   When your goal is to lose weight, you must eat less than 1,200 calories per day. Be aware of what are you eating. Write it down. Add it up.

Persevere   Effort matters. Success and failure have their turn. Get back on the horse.

Herbal Treatments   Chinese herb stores abound with weight loss products. Most are digestive aids that combine herbs to transform phlegm with herbs to promote digestion with other herbs to promote diuresis and elimination. The best known of these is Bojenmi Tea, which is widely available in teabags and as loose tea. The product has a pleasant taste and is steeped as tea.

We reccommend the following two formulas to aid dieters
More Energy from Less Food Powder   No matter what kind of diet you are on, this formula can result in better digestion and potentially lower food requirements. It uses equal amounts of the following combined herbs.

> *Crataegus (shan za)*
> *Aurantium fructus (zhi ke)*
> *Zingiberis radix (sheng jiang)*
> *Perilla folium (zi su ye)*
> *Pogostemon herba (huo xiang)*
> *Citrus pericarpium (chen pi)*
> *Raphanus semen (lai fu zi)*

If taken as powder or granules, take three grams before each meal
Ruin Your Appetite Powder   This combination of herbs reduces appetite by lifting the Qi, causing a sensation of fullness in the stomach. It could upset your stomach, so it is not recommended for those with digestive problems. It can be used for courses of four months or less. It uses equal amounts of the following herbs.

> *Platycodi (ji geng)*
> *Notopterygium (qiang huo)*
> *Bupleurum (chai hu)*
> *Astragalus (huang qi)*
> *Cimicifugia (sheng ma)*

Zoster and Other Viruses

Herbal Treatment   Chinese herbs don't kill viruses, but they can make them impotent. Reproductive rates of viruses like herpes zoster, herpes simplex, and many of their microbial relatives can be lowered by using the right herbal mixtures (see the Cold and Flu section of this chapter).

Herpes Zoster shingles and chicken pox

Herbs to Ingest *Xiao feng wan*: many brands available; *Lian chiao pai tu pian*: Tianjin brand; *Chuan xin lian* (antiphlogistic pills): United, Plum Flower, Guangdong brands; *Ching re chieh tu* herbal beverage: Tianjin brand

Herbs to Apply Topically *Topical medicine #1:* Mash together and apply to affected area:

Aloes herba	*lu hui*	aloe	1 fresh leaf
Borneol	*Bin pien*	Borneol camphor	1 gram
Margarite	*zhen zhu*	pearl	1 gram

Topical medicine #2: Combine herbs with two cups of sesame oil and fry until herbs are brown. Strain oil and cool for a few minutes, then combine oil with 120 grams of beeswax. Apply topically as needed:

Coptis chinensis	*huang lian*	golden thread	9 grams
Angelica sinenses	*dang gui*	*tang kwei*	15 grams
Phellodendron amurense	*huang bai*	amur cork tree	9 grams
Rehmannia glutinosa	*sheng di*	raw foxglove root	30 grams
Curcuma longa	*jiang huang*	turmeric rhizome	9 grams

Herpes Simplex genital and oral herpes

Herbs to Ingest *Long dan xie gan wan,* for genital herpes (many brands available); *Lian Chiao Cheh Tu Pian*: for oral or facial herpes, Tienjin brand

Herbs to Apply Topically *Watermelon Frost* (a spray powder made by United Manufactory in Guangdong); *Superior Sore Throat powder* made by Meizhou and Fitshan

7

Herbs and Their Categories

erbs are categorized by the action or function they perform. An herb may have several different uses; however, it is categorized under only one. The secondary actions are noted in the description of the herb. There are eighteen major categories of action. Several subcategories encompass thousands of medicinal substances. This chapter lists primary categories and subcategories, and the more popular or interesting herbs. One or two herbs in each category are described in detail and others are referenced. A few of these substances are rare and remarkably exotic. Some are plants unfamiliar to Americans. But many herbs are commonplace, ingredients you might find in your kitchen, sweep off your porch, or find in your garden. Each herb in this chapter is identified by its Chinese medicinal, English, and botanical (usually Latin) names. For reference in the dosage sections, grams are a common unit of measure for herbs; a gram is one twenty-eighth of an ounce.

Herbs That Release Exterior Conditions

This category of herbs treats conditions that are considered superficial and that generally reside on the surface of the body. They are used to treat colds, flu, and similar respiratory diseases, addressing symptoms such as fever, chills, headache, stiff neck, body aches, and nasal congestion. Almost all herbs in this group are considered diaphoretics (increase sweating). Sweating, considered therapeutic, assists the body to expel pathogens straight through the skin. This category is divided into two subgroups: Warm Pungent Herbs for Releasing the Exterior (cold conditions) and Cool Pungent Herbs for Releasing the Exterior (hot conditions). Hot and cold conditions are distinguished by several diagnostic observations, including the pulse, the severity of fever, and other symptoms.

Warm Pungent Herbs for Releasing the Exterior

Ma Huang (Ephedra, *Herba ephedra*)

Properties According to Chinese Medicine Pungent and bitter taste, warm temperature

Clinical Functions *Ma huang* releases exterior, disperses cold, circulates lung Qi, promotes urination

Part of Plant Used Stem

Cautions and Contraindications *Ma huang* can cause excess stimulation to the heart, restlessness, and tremors, and raise blood pressure. Do not use for patients whose bodies are weak or deficient. Overdoses can result in excessive sweating, raised blood pressure, rapid heartbeat, tremors, and restlessness. *Ma huang* has been misused as a stimulant and weight loss drug. It is not recommended during pregnancy or for those with high blood pressure. Do not exceed recommended dosage.

Daily Dosage and Administration Boiled whole: three to nine grams; powdered: one gram is considered safe. However, be careful to not take more of this herb. The honey-roasted version of *ma huang* is considered milder, with fewer harsh effects.

Notes *Ma huang* is an amazingly useful herb. It is also the source of ephedrine (amphetamine), a drug that will likely be regulated similarly to coca, opium, and cannabis. Herbs with both medicinal and potentially harmful recreational uses have been classified as dangerous by U.S. federal authorities. The Food and Drug Administration has restricted their use. Because "restriction" means "prohibited," these herbs become freely available for recreational use via the underground economy. Unfortunately, the recreational abuse causes their medical uses to be severely curtailed.

Ma huang is a useful and medicinal herb because it facilitates the circulation of lung Qi, reduces wheezing, promotes urination, and reduces edema. It can be used with cinnamon twigs (*gui zhi, Ramulus cinnamomi*) and other herbs for treatment of the common cold, cough, asthma, and other respiratory ills. When this herb was more readily available, it helped many of my patients avoid inhalers and steroids.

Until the December 2003 ban by the FDA, ephedrine extracted from *ma huang* was a key ingredient in many modern cold remedies, such as Sudafed®, which were easily abused as an amphetamine. This is a prime example of how whole herbs work better and are safer than their pharmaceutical cousins.

Other Herbs in This Category
Cinnamon twigs: *gui zhi, Cinnamomi cassia ramulus*
Perilla leaf: *su ye, Perilla frutescentis folium*
Fresh ginger: *sheng jiang, Zingiberis officinalis rhizoma*
Wild ginger root: *xi xin, Asari cum radice herba*
Scallion (green onion): *cong bai, Allii fistulosi herba*

Cool Pungent Herbs for Releasing the Exterior

Ge Gen (Kudzu root, *Pueraria radix*) and **Ge Hua** (Kudzu flower, *Pueraria flos)*

Properties of Chinese Medicine Sweet, pungent taste, cool temperature

Clinical Functions Kudzu root and flower, *ge gen* and *ge hua*, release the muscles, nourish fluids, bring rash to the surface, and alleviate diarrhea.

Part of Plant Used Root or flower

Cautions and Contraindications None

Daily Dosage and Administration Boiled whole herbs: six to nine grams; for alcoholism: fifteen grams. Powdered: one to two grams daily; for alcoholism: three to six grams.

Notes Kudzu root is traditionally used to release the muscles of the neck and shoulders when a cold or flu causes pain and stiffness. It is found in numerous formulas to treat upper body pain and certain headaches. Kudzu has become widely used throughout Asia to effectively treat alcoholism. But its true medicinal gifts are unknown to most Americans; it is considered a noxious weed that is displacing the natural flora of Georgia and much of the South.

Chai Hu (Hare's ear root, *Bupleurum radix*)

Properties of Chinese Medicine Bitter and slightly acrid taste, cool temperature

Clinical Functions *Chai hu* relaxes constrained liver Qi, raises yang Qi

Part of Plant Used Root

Cautions and Contraindications *Chai hu* can be slightly drying when used alone or over long periods of time. Do not use with dry cough from lung yin deficiency or with headache caused by liver fire rising. *Chai hu* can occasionally cause nausea.

Daily Dosage and Administration Boiled: three to twelve grams; powdered: one-half to three grams

Notes *Chai hu* has two main functions and is always used in a formula with other herbs, most often with white peony root, which helps to moisten and offset the herb's drying side effect. Use *chai hu* with mint or mimosa bark to circulate the Qi of the chest to relieve depression, PMS, and the effects of stress on the body (see *hsiao yao wan* in Chapter 5, "Famous Herbal Medicines").

Chai hu also raises the Qi and is one of the three main herbs used to lift fallen organs. The others are black cohosh (*sheng ma*) and *Astragalus* (*huang qi*). These herbs are often used together when the Qi has lost its lifting quality and resulted in conditions such as uterine prolapse, anal prolapse, varicose veins, and some cases of hemorrhoids.

Other Herbs in This Category
Peppermint: *bo he, Mentha herba*
Cicada moulting: *chan tui, Cicadae periiostracum*
Chrysanthemum flower: *ju hua, Chrysanthemi morifoli flos*
Fermented soy bean: *dan dou chi, Soja praeparatum semen*

Herbs That Clear Heat

This huge category consists of herbs that treat febrile conditions as well as any condition with "heat" signs. These include rapid pulse, dry or sore throat, red face, red eyes, hot flashes, dark urine, irritability, and constipation or dry stool. In clinical terms, many of these herbs have anti-inflammatory and antibiotic effects. Categories are Herbs That Clear Heat and Dry Dampness, Herbs that Clear Heat and Clean Toxins, Herbs that Clear Heat and Relieve Summer Heat, and Herbs That Clear Heat and Cool the Blood (Quell Fire). The herbs in this last subcategory are quite cold and are used to treat high fevers and the thirst and delirium that can accompany them.

Zhi Zi (Gardenia, *Fructus gardenia jasminoidis*)

Properties of Chinese Medicine Bitter taste, cold temperature

Clinical Functions Zhi zi clears heat and relieves irritability, drains damp heat, cools blood, stops bleeding, and reduces swelling from trauma

Part of Plant Used Fruit

Cautions and Contraindications Zhi zi is contraindicated in patients with loose stool or diarrhea due to spleen deficiency cold

Daily Dosage and Administration Boiled: six to twelve grams; powdered: one to two grams, charred and applied topically to stop bleeding

Notes Gardenia seeds, *zhi zi*, are one of the best herbs for clearing heat from the heart. They are thus used in formulas designed for insomnia, irritability, restlessness, and other symptoms of heart fire. Use zhi zi together with gypsum (*shi gao*) for fevers with thirst. Combine it with raw foxglove root (*sheng di huang*) for mouth or tongue sores, or reduced urination due to heat in the heart channel.

Other Herbs in This Category
Gypsum: *shi gao*
Anemarrhena root: *zhi mu*
Bat feces: *ye ming sha, Vespertili excrementum*

Herbs That Clear Heat and Cool the Blood

"Blood heat" occurs when infectious diseases or other forms of heat enter the blood. This can produce rashes, nosebleeds, spitting or coughing up blood, and hemorrhages. For these conditions, herbs that clear heat and cool the blood are combined with herbs that stop bleeding.

Sheng Di Huang (Raw foxglove root, *Rehmannia radix*)

Properties of Chinese Medicine   Sweet and bitter taste, cold temperature

Clinical Functions   *Sheng di huang* clears heat and cools the blood, nourishes the yin and the blood, generates fluids, and cools heart fire

Part of Plant Used   Root

Cautions and Contraindications   Use *sheng di huang* cautiously in patients with phlegm damp or spleen deficient conditions. Do not use in pregnant women who are blood or spleen deficient.

Daily Dosage and Administration   Boiled: nine to thirty grams; powdered: one to six grams

Notes   It is important to know the difference between raw foxglove root (*sheng di huang*) and cooked foxglove root (*shu di huang*). *Sheng di huang* cools the blood, whereas *shu di huang* tonifies the blood. Even though their subsidiary functions are similar, their medicinal uses are quite different and cannot be automatically substituted for each other. Use *sheng di huang* with glue made of donkey hide (*e jiao*) for nosebleeds stemming from yin deficient heat. Combine with *bai mao gen* for blood in the urine due to heat entering the blood level. Use *sheng di huang* together with *sha ren* (*Fructus ammomi*) to help digestibility and absorption.

Other Herbs in This Category
Tree peony root bark: *mu dan pi, Moutan radicis cortex*
Ningpo figwort root: *xuan shen, Radix scrophularia*
Groomwell root: *zi cao, Radix lithospermi*

Herbs That Clear Heat and Dry Dampness

These herbs are used for "damp heat" patterns that are often combinations of inflammatory or infectious conditions with a discharge of fluid. Herbs from this category are thus used to treat dysentery, boils, weeping, eczema, and other conditions with pus or fluid discharge.

Huang Lian (Golden Thread, *Coptidis rhizoma*)

Properties of Chinese Medicine   Bitter taste, cold temperature

Clinical Functions   Huang lian extinguishes fire and detoxifies fire poisons. Clears heat and drains dampness, heart fire, topical heat, and stomach fire.

Part of plant used   Rhizome

Cautions and Contraindications   *Huang lian* is contraindicated in treating deficiency heat patterns caused by yin deficiency: patients with diarrhea from cold or deficient conditions, and cold stomach. Long-term use of this herb is not advised.

Daily Dosage and Administration   Boiled: three to twelve grams; powdered: one-half to three grams. Can be taken alone or in combination. Use more when using as a single herb. Cooking may reduce potency.

Notes   Some practitioners see *huang lian* as similar to goldenseal, which is also known for its "antibiotic" properties. But neither *huang lian* nor goldenseal kills microorganisms as do pharmaceutical antibiotics. Instead, *huang lian* offers antimicrobial effects proven to inhibit the growth of streptococcus, staphylococcus, and shigella dysenteriae, the bacteria that usually cause dysentery. Studies have shown this herb to be as effective as sulfa drugs in curing bacillary dysentery with no side effects. *Huang lian* has also been shown to be effective for typhoid fever, tuberculosis, scarlet fever, and diphtheria.

Other Herbs in This Category

Skullcap root: *huang Qin, Radix scutellaria*
Dragon gallbladder herb: *long dan cao, Radix gentianae scabrae*
Amur cork tree bark: *huang bai, Cortex phellodendri*

Herbs That Clear Heat and Clean Toxins

These herbs neutralize the toxic effects of bacteria, virus, and other pathogens. They are used for various types of infections, including purulent (runny) sores and abscesses, as well as viral infections.

Jin Yin Hua   (Honeysuckle Flowers, *Flos lonicera japonica*)

Properties of Chinese Medicine   Sweet taste, cold temperature

Clinical Functions   *Jin yin hua* clears heat, detoxifies fire poisons, expels wind heat, and clears damp heat in the lower burner

Part of Plant Used   Flower

Cautions and Contraindications   Do not use *jin yin hua* in cases of diarrhea from spleen deficiency cold

Daily Dosage and Administration   Boiled: nine to fifteen grams; powdered: two to three grams

Notes   *Jin yin hua* is used to expel respiratory infections (wind heat) and also to detoxify fire poisons that may appear as hot painful sores, swellings, or abscesses. It is synergistic and almost always used together with forsythia fruit (*lian Qiao*). This potent anti-viral combination forms the basis of the formula *yin chiao cheh tu pian* (Honeysuckle Forsythia Clean Toxin pill) (see Chapter 6, "Treatments of Ailments A to Z," Cold and Flu).

Other Herbs in This Category

Forsythia fruit: *lian qiao*
Indigo: *ban lan gen*
Dandelion: *pu gong yin*
Puffball: *ma bo*

Herbs That Clear and Relieve Summer Heat

"Summer heat" is an illness that usually, but not always, occurs during the late summer. Fevers, chest discomfort, irritability, diarrhea, sweating, reduced urination, and thirst are characteristic of this condition. Summer heat patterns can be diagnosed as flu, fever with unknown origin, respiratory or urinary tract infection, or heat stroke. The herbs in this category all have diuretic effects, relieve fevers and diarrhea, and generate fluids to dissipate thirst.

He Ye (Lotus Leaf, *Folium nelumbinis*)

Properties of Chinese Medicine Bitter and slightly sweet taste, neutral temperature

Clinical Functions *He ye* relieves fever and diarrhea caused by summer heat, astringes excessive sweating, and stops bleeding caused by heat or stagnation

Part of Plant Used Leaf

Cautions and Contraindications Do not use *he ye* for bleeding caused by excessive cold

Daily Dosage and Administration In formula: nine to fifteen grams; used alone: at least thirty grams

Notes The lotus stem, *lian geng*, can also be used; however, its properties are slightly different. Whereas the leaf *he ye* has its strongest action in the lower burner (organs in the lower body cavity), the lotus stem moves the Qi of the chest, making it more useful for patterns with discomfort in the chest, rather than with diarrhea.

Other Herbs in This Category

Mung bean: *lu dou, Semen phaseoli radiati*
Watermelon fruit: *xi gua, Fructus citrullus vulgaris*
Hyacinth bean: *bian dou, Semen dolichoris lablab*

Herbs That Drain Downward

These herbs fall into three subcategories: purgatives, laxatives, and harsh expellants. Purgatives stimulate or lubricate the intestines. Some, considered harsh purgatives, have strong heat-clearing properties and are used for constipation and other heat-based maladies. Others, moist laxatives, are more mild and used for constipation in the elderly. These are often oil-bearing seeds or nuts. Finally, there are harsh expellants (cathartics). These very strong herbs induce diarrhea or urination. They can produce violent effects and are only used for emergencies.

Purgatives

Da Huang   (Chinese rhubarb rhizome, *Rhei rhizoma*)

Properties of Chinese Medicine   Bitter taste, cold temperature

Clinical Functions   *Da huang* moves stool and drains heat, drains heat from the blood, breaks congealed blood, and detoxifies fire poison

Part of Plant Used   Rhizome

Cautions and Contraindications   Do not use *da huang* during pregnancy, nursing, or postpartum. Patients with loose stools should not use this herb. Use cautiously for patients whose systems are weak or deficient.

Daily Dosage and Administration   Boiled: three to six grams, boiled no longer than ten minutes; powdered: one-half to one gram in formulas. It may also be applied topically for burns or inflamed skin lesions.

Notes   Marco Polo went to China in search of da huang. During this era, constipation was rampant due to diets lacking in fresh fruits and vegetables. When Marco Polo brought the legendary herb back from China, it proved superior to anything being used in Europe. It did not take long before everyone knew about Chinese rhubarb for constipation. *Da huang* became the most sought-after medicine of its time, and was a big reason for East-West trade for about a thousand years.

Note that overcooked rhubarb can have an astringent, binding effect, the opposite of the desired effect, so it is important to either use the raw herb or cook it for fewer than ten minutes. Like any strong downward-draining herb, Chinese rhubarb root, not the same as rhubarb that you'd buy in the market, should not be used during pregnancy.

Other Herbs in This Category
Epsom salts: *mang xiao, Mirabilitum*
Senna leaf: *fang xie ye, Folium sennae*
Aloe juice: *lu hui, Herba aloes*

Moist Laxatives

These herbs are much less harsh than the purgatives. They are chiefly oil-bearing seeds or nuts, and achieve their laxative effect by moistening the intestines. They are often used in combination with other herbs to treat constipation arising from deficient blood or yin.

Huo Ma Ren (Marijuana seeds, *Cannabis sativa semen*)

Properties of Chinese Medicine Sweet taste, neutral temperature

Clinical Functions *Huo ma ren* nourishes and moistens the intestines, and promotes the healing of sores

Part of Plant Used Seed

Cautions and Contraindications *Huo ma ren* is not recommended for long-term use, which can cause kidney deficiency

Daily Dosage and Administration Like all other oil-bearing seeds, it must be ground with mortar and pestle before use. Boiled: three to nine grams; powdered: one-half to one gram.

Notes Though they have no hallucinogenic effect and have been boiled so they will not grow, marijuana seeds (*huo ma ren*) are often available from importers though they are still illegal in the United States. Since these seeds have been cultivated for their oil, not for their hallucinogenic effect, even if they did grow, the resulting plant would likely be useless to pot smokers. Current law listing marijuana as a dangerous drug does a major disservice to the public, as this herb has important and well-documented benefits.

Other Herbs in This Category
Bush cherry pit: *yu li ren, Semen pruni*

Harsh Cathartics

Qian Niu Zi (Morning Glory Seeds, *Pharbitides semen*)

Properties of Chinese Medicine Poisonous. Bitter and acrid taste, cold temperature.

Clinical Functions *Qian niu zi* expels water, phlegm, parasites, and congested fluids

Part of Plant Used Seeds

Cautions and Contraindications *Qian niu* zi is contraindicated for pregnancy and nursing, and for weak or deficient people. Overdose can cause nausea, vomiting, hallucinations, and blood in the urine.

Daily Dosage and Administration Four and a half to nine grams in decoction; one-half to two grams when used as a powder or taken alone

Notes *Qian niu zi* has been used as a hallucinogenic drug. It is best used for ascites or edema, or together with *xing ren* (almond kernel) and *ting li zi* (woods whitlow seed) for wheezing, and to relieve the sense of fullness in the chest caused by congested fluids. *Qian niu zi* is used with *bing lan* (betel nut) to expel parasites.

Other Herbs in This Category

Gan sui, Radix euphorbiae
Daphne flower: *yuan hua, Flos daphnes genkwa*
Woods whitlow grass seed: *ting li zi, Semen tinglizi*

Herbs That Drain Dampness

These are rather gentle herbs, not harsh cathartics. They help escort water out of the tissue and away from the body. They are used in formulas for edema (swelling), primarily in the lower extremities. They are also used in formulas designed to break down and remove phlegm or water from the body, and also to treat congested fluids, fluids that obstruct flow, producing respiratory, digestive, or other problems.

Fu Lin (Hoelen mushroom, *Poria cocos*)

Properties of Chinese Medicine Sweet and bland taste, neutral temperature

Clinical Functions *Fu ling* promotes urination and leaches dampness from the tissues. It strengthens the spleen, transforms phlegm, quiets the heart, and calms the spirit.

Part of Plant Used Fruiting body

Cautions and Contraindications *Fu ling* is not for patients who have excessive urine volume

Daily Dosage and Administration Boiled: nine to ninety grams; powdered: one to four grams

Notes This common fungus usually grows on fallen pine trees. *Fu ling* has a mild nature and is combined with other herbs (not used alone) to smooth out their rough effects within a formula. This herb drains dampness. Though not a strong diuretic, it helps leach water from the tissues, and is used in many formulas that require mild diuretic action. *Fu ling* is also a mild spleen tonic and is used in cases of deficient spleen and dampness with symptoms of loss of appetite, phlegm in the lungs, and diarrhea.

Jin Qian Cao (Gold Coin Herb, also known as glechoma when from Jiangsu Province, desmodium when from Guangdong Province, and lysimachia when from Sichuan Province)

Part of Plant Used Entire plant

Properties of Chinese Medicine Jiangsu glechoma has a bitter, acrid taste, and a cool temperature; Guandong desmodium has a sweet, bland taste, and a neutal temperature; Sichuan lysimachia has a salty taste and a neutral temperature.

Clinical Functions *Jin qian cao* expels stones, promotes urination, detoxifies poisons, and reduces swellings

Cautions and Contraindications Large doses of *jin qian cao* taken over long periods of time have been suspected of causing electrolyte depletion that led to dizziness and heart palpitations

Daily Dosage and Administration Boiled: fifteen to thirty grams; powdered: three to six grams

Notes These different plants from various parts of China are designated as the same herb due to one defining healing property: they all expel stones. *Jin qian cao* is combined with *hula shi* (talc) or *yu mi xu* (corn silk) to expel kidney stones. Combine it with *yin chen* (artemesia capillaries), *chai hu* (hare's ear root), and *zhi zi* (gardenia seeds) for gallstones.

Other Herbs in This Category
Talc: *hua shi*, talcum
Seeds of Job's tears: *yi yi ren, Coicis lachryma semen*
Plantago seeds: *che qian zi, Plantaginis semen*

Corn silk: *yu mi xu, Stylus zeae mays*
Artemesia, young shoots: *yin chen, Herba artemesiae*

Herbs That Expel Wind and Damp from the Surface

These herbs are used to relieve pain in the muscles, tendons, joints, and bones. Primarily they are used for a condition known as Painful Obstruction (Bi Syndrome), where a weakness in the body's defensive energy (*wei Qi*) allows the incursion of atmospheric influences such as Wind, Cold, Hot, or Damp Painful Obstructions. This condition is commonly called arthritis.

Wu Jia Pi (Siberian ginseng, *Cortex radices—Acanthopanax gracilistylus, Acanthopanax sessiliflourus, Acanthopanax senticosus*. All three species are used.)

Properties of Chinese Medicine Spicy taste, warm temperature

Clinical Functions *Wu jia pi* expels wind damp, strengthens the sinews and bones, and reduces swelling

Part of Plant Used Bark of the root

Cautions and Contraindications Use *wu jia pi* cautiously in people who exhibit yin deficient heat signs.

Daily Dosage and Administration Boiled: four and a half to nine grams; powdered: one to two grams

Notes Most natural food stores sell Siberian ginseng as ginseng (*ren shen*), which is incorrect. It is a distant and inexpensive relative without the energy building, renewing properties of *ren shen*. Practitioners use only the bark of the root of this common plant to expel wind dampness from the joints, tendons, and bones. Best for chronic osteoarthritic conditions caused by deficiency, it is useful in restoring the smooth flow of Qi and relieving pain, especially in the elderly. The herb also transforms dampness to reduce swelling, and is used together with *du huo* for edema, and for leg pain that may involve internal swelling that is not visible on the outside. This painful condition is called Damp Leg Qi.

Cang Er Zi (Cocklebur Fruit, *Fructus xanthium*)

Properties of Chinese Medicine Poisonous. Sweet and bitter taste, warm temperature

Clinical Functions *Cang er zi* unblocks the nasal passages and expels wind and dampness from the skin

Part of Plant Used Fruit

Cautions and Contraindications Do not use *cang er zi* for headaches caused by deficient blood

Daily Dosage and Administration *Cang er zi* is slightly poisonous in its raw form; cooking neutralizes the toxin. Boiled: four and a half to nine grams. Do not use as a milled powder. Water-extracted granules are acceptable.

Notes *Cang er zi* is unique in this category for expelling wind from the skin. It is used for nasal congestion, headache, and itching, making it useful for mollifying allergic sensitivity. You can find it in many allergy-related formulas. This herb is slightly poisonous when used raw. Heating or cooking it eliminates the toxicity. Use *cang er zi* with *bai ji li* (*Tribuli territories*) to make an external wash to relieve itching. Combine it with *xin ye hua* (magnolia buds) for nasal congestion, and with *wu wei zi* (*schisandra*) for allergic rhinitis.

Other Herbs in This Category
Duhuo root: *du huo, Angelica pubescens*
Snake skin: *she tui, Serpentis periostracum*
Mulberry twigs: *sang zhi, Mori alba ramulus*

Herbs That Transform Phlegm and Stop Coughing

This group is divided into Herbs to Transform Hot Phlegm and Herbs to Transform Cold Phlegm. Herbs that treat hot phlegm are used mainly for coughs caused by thick, dry, or difficult-to-expectorate phlegm that has been reduced and thickened by heat. Some of these herbs are also used for goiter, others for convulsions or psychosis caused by Hot Phlegm Obstructing the Heart Orifice. They are considered an expectorant, and are anti-tussive (relieves cough), anti-inflammatory, and sedative in their effects.

Herbs to Transform Hot Phlegm

Hai Zao   (Seaweed, *Sargassi herba*)

Properties of Chinese Medicine   Bitter and salty taste, cold temperature

Clinical Functions   *Hai zao* clears heat and reduces neck nodules; it directs the action of other herbs to the neck and throat, and relieves hernial pain

Part of Plant Used   Entire plant

Cautions and Contraindications   Use *hai zao* cautiously in people with weak digestion. It is traditionally considered incompatible with *gan cao* (licorice root).

Daily Dosage and Administration   Boiled: four and a half to fifteen grams; powdered: one to three grams

Notes   *Hai zao* (seaweed) is a part of most formulas used to treat goiter, scrofula, and thyroid conditions. Its high iodine content serves to supplement the deficient iodine characteristic of several thyroid conditions. The iodine contained in seaweed is very slow to metabolize, and is therefore not considered toxic as pure iodine. Though seaweed is considered incompatible with licorice root, according to historical Chinese medical texts, the combination has been well established as safe in neck nodule and thyroid formulas.

Other Herbs in This Category
Dried bamboo sap: *zhu li, Bambusa succus*
Bamboo shavings: *zhu ru, Bambusa in taeniis*
Kelp: *kun bu, Thallus algae*

Herbs to Transform Cold Phlegm

This class of herbs is used for Cold or Damp Phlegm marked by thin, frothy, or watery sputum. Some of these herbs are also used to treat phlegm obstructing the channels. These reduce nodules and other phlegm obstructions that might block flow and cause symptoms of numbness, facial pain, paralysis, and other signs we associate with Wind Stroke (stroke). Several of these herbs are quite strong and have a harsh, toxic nature. They should be used with caution.

Ban Xia (*Pinellia, Pinellia ternata, Rhizoma preperatum*)

Properties of Chinese Medicine Poisonous. Acrid taste, warm temperature.

Clinical Functions Ban xia dries dampness and transforms phlegm; it causes rebellious Qi to descend, harmonizes the stomach to stop vomiting, and dissipates nodules.

Part of Plant Used Rhizome

Cautions and Contraindications Ban xia in its raw form is poisonous. Only processed *Rhizoma pinellia* is safe to use. It is rendered non-toxic through deep-frying with ginger or alum. Symptoms of poisoning can include burning and numbness in the lips and throat, nausea, and pressure in the chest. The antidote is raw ginger. Contraindicated in all cases of bleeding. Do not use for dry cough. Use cautiously in heat conditions with fever or infection. Not recommended in combination with *wu tou* (*Radix aconite*).

Daily Dosage and Administration Cooked (deep-fried): four and a half to twelve grams; raw: *ban xia* is only used topically for skin ulcerations and carbuncles.

Notes Ban xia must be prepared properly before use: it must be detoxified by deep frying with other substances, such as sugar, ginger, alum, or vinegar, which also can help bring out particular properties. It is usually available only in these forms. *Ban xia* is a very useful herb; it dries dampness, transforms phlegm, and causes rebellious Qi to descend. *Ban xia* also harmonizes the stomach and stops vomiting. These properties make it one of the most effective substances to control nausea. Combined with *chen pi* (aged tangerine peel) and *huo xiang* (patchouli), it can instantly relieve coughs caused by thin, watery sputum affecting the lungs. It is also one of the main herbs used to dissipate neck nodules for sufferers of goiter and scrofula. For this purpose, *ban xia* is best combined with *hai zao* (seaweed) or *kun bu* (kelp).

Other Herbs in This Category
Balloon flower root: *jie geng, Platycodi grandiflori radix*
Jack-in-the-pulpit rhizome: *tian nan xing, Rhizoma arisaemati*s
White mustard seed: *bai ji zi, Semen sinapis albae*

Herbs That Relieve Coughing and Wheezing

Coughing and wheezing are regarded as branch (visible) symptoms of root (invisible) conditions. Thus, these herbs are combined with other herbs designed to treat the underlying root of the particular condition.

Pi Pa Ye (Loquat Leaf, *Eriobotrya folium*)

Properties of Chinese Medicine Bitter, cool taste and temperature

Clinical Functions *Pi pa ye* moistens the lungs, expels phlegm, clears lung heat, and redirects lung and stomach Qi downward

Part of Plant Used Leaf

Cautions and Contraindications Do not use *pi pa ye* when vomiting is caused by cold stomach, or when cough is caused by cold in the lungs

Daily Dosage and Administration Boiled: four and a half to twelve grams of dried herbs, or thirty to fifty grams of fresh leaves; powdered: one to three grams. Be sure to clean fresh leaves of "hair" to prevent throat irritation.

Notes Use *pi pa ye* (loquat leaf) together with *xing ren* (almond kernel) for non-productive coughs accompanied by fever and dry throat, or for coughs with thick sputum that is difficult to expectorate. Use *pi pa ye* with *lu gen* (reed rhizome) for vomiting that results from a febrile disease that has caused injury to the fluids. Add *bai mao gen* for vomiting blood from such injuries. Toast this herb with honey to enhance its fluid-generating properties. Toast *pi pa ye* with ginger to increase its ability to reduce nausea.

Other Herbs in This Category
Purple perilla fruit: *su zi, Perillia frutescentis fructus*
Almond kernel: *xing ren, Pruni armeniaca semen*
Purple aster root: *zi wan, Asteris tatarici radix*

Herbs That Transform Dampness

Herbs that transform dampness reduce fluids in the Middle Burner (in the middle body cavity that contains the liver, spleen, and stomach). Symptoms of excessive dampness in your middle burner are pressure, bloating, or a feeling of uncomfortable fullness in the abdomen, nausea or vomiting, loss of appetite, and diarrhea, often with difficulty defecating. Since these herbs tend to reduce fluids, they must be used cautiously in people whose systems tend to be dry (yin deficient or blood deficient).

Huo Xiang (Patchouli, *Herba agastaches seu pogostemi*)

Properties of Chinese Medicine Acrid taste, slightly warm temperature

Clinical Functions *Huo xiang* transforms dampness caused by spleen deficiency, harmonizes the middle burner, stops vomiting, and releases the exterior to expel dampness

Part of Plant Used Entire plant

Cautions and Contraindications Do not use *huo xiang* with deficient yin heat signs such as night sweats, chronic sore throat, or mild persistent flu-like fevers and symptoms. Do not use in cases of heartburn due to stomach fire.

Daily Dosage and Administration Boiled: four and a half to twelve grams when boiled in decoction. Do not boil more than fifteen minutes or important volatile components will evaporate. Powdered: one to two grams in formula with other herbs.

Notes *Huo xiang* relieves damp conditions that exist both on the surface of and deep inside the body. This makes it the optimal choice to use when exterior pathogens, like cold or flu, cause damp symptoms such as nasal congestion, and penetrate deeper into the body, producing nausea, vomiting, bloating, or stomachache. Sometimes these conditions are referred to as Summer Colds. In general, combine *huo xiang* with *ban xia* for nausea and vomiting. However, for nausea from morning sickness, it's best combined with *sha ren*, (*Amomi villosum semen seu fructus*), which has a beneficial effect on the fetus.

Other Herbs in This Category
Magnolia bark: *hou po, Magnolia officinalis cortex*
Cardamon: *bai dou kou, Amomi cardamomi fructus*
Grains of paradise: *sha ren, Amomi villosum semen seu fructus*

Herbs That Relieve Food Stagnation

Food and digestate normally flow downward. When food flow is constrained in the stomach due to improper eating events or habits, the result is food stagnation. It can appear as abdominal bloating, stomach pain, belching, sour taste, or even diarrhea. Commonly referred to as indigestion, food stagnation often results from overeating, irregular food consumption, or eating under duress.

Herbs used for food stagnation are not all alike. Though they all relieve the primary symptoms, they have different secondary effects. *Lai fu zi* (radish seed) also causes the Qi to descend, so is also useful for chronic productive cough with wheezing. *Ji nei jin* (chicken gizzard lining) is also a kidney tonic used for bed-wetting and for kidney stones. *Shan za* (hawthorn berry) also transforms congealed blood and dissipates masses, is used for angina and other heart pain, and has also been shown to significantly reduce cholesterol.

Shan Za   (Hawthorn Berry, *Crataegi fructus*)

Properties of Chinese Medicine   Sour and sweet taste, slightly warm temperature

Clinical Functions   *Shan za* dissolves food and reduces stagnation, transforms congealed blood and dissipates masses, and alleviates diarrhea

Part of Plant Used   Fruit

Cautions and Contraindications   Use *shan za* cautiously in people with acid regurgitation

Daily Dosage and Administration   Boiled: six to twelve grams; powdered: one to three grams. Ripe fruit dissolves food stagnation. Unripe fruit stops diarrhea. Charred fruit is used for dysentery with bleeding.

Notes   When you eat several hawthorn candy wafers after a big Thanksgiving dinner, you will likely be hungry for desert within a few minutes.

This herb also has healthier uses. *Shan za*, hawthorn fruit, has been used since the fourteenth century to relieve meat accumulations that cause abdominal bloating, pain, or diarrhea. This herb has also been shown to reduce serum cholesterol. *Shan za* is also potentially useful in the prevention and treatment of heart and artery diseases.

Other Herbs in This Category
Radish seed: *lai fu zi, Raphani sativi semen*
Chicken gizzard: *ji nei jin, Endithelium corneum gigeraia galli*
Barley sprouts: *mai ya, Fructus hordei germenantus*
Rice sprouts: *gu ya, Fructus orzya germanantus*

Herbs That Regulate the Qi

Qi problems come in three basic types: Deficient Qi, Stagnant Qi, and Rebellious Qi. Herbs in this category all move or regulate the Qi. They address stagnation and are usually combined with tonifying (strengthening) herbs such as *ren shen* (ginseng) or *huang qi* (Astragalus) to treat deficient Qi, and also with directional herbs such as *chuan xiong* (Liguisticum) for upward Qi redirection, or *niu xi* (Achyranthes) for downward Qi redirection.

Chen Pi   (Aged tangerine peel, *Pericarpium citri reticulatae*)

Properties of Chinese Medicine   Acrid and bitter taste, warm temperature, aromatic smell

Clinical Functions   *Chen pi* moves the Qi of the lung and stomach, strengthens the spleen, directs Qi downward, dries dampness, and transforms phlegm. *Chen pi* is used as an adjuvant to herbs that cause stagnation.

Cautions and Contraindications   *Chen pi* is not for dry cough caused by heat or deficient yin

Part of Plant Used   Peel

Daily Dosage and Administration   Boiled: three to nine grams, boiled for less than three minutes. When used in formula, citrus peel should be added at the very end of the boiling. Powdered: one-half to two grams.

Notes   Use aged tangerine peel for abdominal bloating, poor appetite, and nausea and vomiting caused by spleen deficiency or stagnant stomach Qi. Use *chen pi* as an adjuvant in a formula to counteract the stagnating effects of heavy tonifying herbs. A rule of formula-building is that when you build Qi, you must also move Qi; if not, stagnation will occur.

Aged citrus peel imported from China can come from many different orange-like plants, including tangerines and mandarin oranges. You can easily make *chen pi* yourself. Instead of discarding your citrus peels, wash off possible pesticides from the surface, then air-dry them indoors or in shade. After they've dried out, store them in a paper bag. Old is good. The older they are, the better they get.

You can also use fresh citrus peel to relieve nausea. Shave a small piece of citrus peel. When the peel is bent or folded, a tiny spray will puff from the surface. Hold a sliver of peel under your nose, squeeze it, and inhale deeply, breathing in the little spray. Repeat this procedure several times.

Other Herbs in This Category

Immature bitter orange peel: *zi shi, Fructus aurantium*
Buddha hands: *fo shou, Fructus citri sarcodactylis*
Rose petals: *mei gui hua, Flos rosea rugosae*
Lychee nut: *li zhi he, Semen litchi chinensis*
Sandalwood: *tan xiang, Lignum santali albi*

Herbs That Regulate the Blood

There are subcategories of herbs that regulate the blood: Herbs to Nourish the Blood, Herbs to Move the Blood, and Herbs to Stop Bleeding.

Herbs That Nourish the Blood

Dang Gui   (Tangkuei root, *Angelica sinensis*)

Properties of Chinese Medicine   Sweet, acrid, and bitter taste, warm temperature

Clinical Functions   *Dang gui* tonifies the blood, regulates the menses, and invigorates and harmonizes the blood. It also moistens the intestines and moves the stool.

Part of Plant Used Root

Cautions and Contraindications *Dang gui* is contraindicated in people with diarrhea unless modified by the addition of herbs to counteract its laxative effect. The same is true for use with yin deficient patients with heat signs. The warming property of *dang gui* must be modified in these cases by the addition of cooling herbs.

Daily Dosage and Administration Boiled: three to fifteen grams; powdered: one half to three grams. Frying in vinegar boosts its blood-moving properties.

Notes This popular herb is used to benefit the blood (nourish the tissue). The herbalist's axiom is "When you build the blood, you must also move the blood." Forget to move the blood, and you may wind up with stagnation and pain. *Dang gui* is convenient in that it both builds the blood and moves the blood, doing the work of two different herbs. However, *dang gui* should not be used alone, as its laxative properties must usually be checked by other herbs. Probably the most popular formula containing *dang gui* is *ba zhen wan* (see Chapter 5, "Famous Herbal Medicines").

Dang gui and other blood tonics are especially useful for women of child-bearing age who eat little or no red meat. This formula is used in many cases of infertility where blood deficiency is a known cause.

Other Herbs in This Category

Foxglove root, cooked: *shu di huang, Radix rehmanniae*
White peony root: *bai shao, Radix paeonia lactiflora*
Fo ti: *he shou wu, Radix polyfoni multiflori*
Goji berry: *gou qi zi, Fructus lycii chinensis*

Herbs That Vitalize the Blood

Where there is flow, there is no pain. The free flow of blood is vital to health and existence. The circulation system provides nourishment to the body's cells, transports wastes, and helps to cool metabolic heat. When blood flow is challenged, pain is the alarm.

When an herb is known to relieve pain, it is said to have the property of Vitalizing the Blood. Herbs in this category all vitalize the blood, and are almost all used to treat pain. They differ from one another in terms of their strength, where in the body they work best, and other subsidiary effects.

Hong Hua   (Safflower, *Carthami tinctori flo*)

Properties of Chinese Medicine   Acrid taste, warm temperature

Clinical Functions   *Hong hua* invigorates the blood, dispels congealed blood, and aleviates pain

Part of Plant Used   Flower

Cautions and Contraindications   *Hong hua* is not recommended during pregnancy.

Daily Dosage and Administration   Boiled: three to nine grams; powdered: one-half to two grams

Notes   *Hong hua* (safflower) is commonly used for menstrual disorders like dysmenorrhea (painful periods), amenorrhea (no periods), and abdominal masses or tumors. It is also used extensively for pain from injury due to congealed blood. For both these purposes, it is usually combined with *tao ren* (peach kernel). Combining the two creates a srong synergistic effect.

Other Herbs in This Category

Peach seeds: *tao ren, Persica semen*
Szechuan lovage root: *chuan xiong, Ligustici wallichii radix*
Chinese sage root: *dan shen, Salvia miltiorrhiza radix*
Tumeric tuber: *yu jin, Curcuma longa tuber*
Red peony root: *chi shao,Paeonia rubra radix*
Frankincense: *ru xiang, Olibanum gummi*
Myrrh: *mo yao, Commiphora myrrha*

Herbs to Stop Bleeding

While all the herbs in this group stop bleeding, different herbs are used for different conditions. *Ai ye* is warming and is used for bleeding associated with cold conditions. Heat induced bleeding requires cooling herbs such as *ce bai ye*. These herbs are often combined with blood cooling herbs to treat the kind of bleeding known as Reckless Marauding of Hot Blood. They are combined with yin strengthening herbs to treat bleeding patterns associated with yin deficiency heat. Burning (carbonizing) any herb will strengthen its ability to stop bleeding. Stop Bleeding herbs are generally used with caution over short periods of time, because they can cause stagnation of fluids. The following is one notable exception.

Tienchi or Tian qi or San qsi   (Pseudoginseng root, Pseudoginsing, or Notoginseng)

Properties of Chinese Medicine   Sweet and slightly bitter taste, slightly warm temperature

Clinical Functions   *Tienchi* stops bleeding, transforms congealed blood, reduces swelling, and alleviates pain

Part of Plant Used   Root

Cautions and Contraindications   Contraindicated during pregnancy. Use cautiously in people with deficient blood.

Daily Dosage and Administration   Boiled: three to nine grams; powdered: one-third to two grams. Also used topically to stop bleeding.

Notes   Nearly every Chinese citizen knows about this remarkable root, yet few in the West are familiar with it. Used to stop both internal and external bleeding problems, *tienchi* appears to work in a unique way. All other Stop Bleeding herbs promote coagulation and can thus cause stagnation when overused. *Tienchi* appears to stop bleeding without promoting coagulation. This effect may be due to its beneficial effect on the liver. Because it can't cause stagnation, *tienchi* can be safely used for extended periods of time, which makes it indispensable for chronic or recurrent bleeding conditions.

Though it is classified as a Stop Bleeding herb, *tienchi* has the oddly paradoxical function of moving the blood, thus relieving pain, particularly pain from injury and trauma. This unique herb moves the blood and stops bleeding, both at the same time.

Because it moves the blood, *tienchi* also reduces swelling. Other successful uses for *tienchi* include treatment for trauma, most bleeding problems, angina, and the pain of Crohn's disease. The flower of this plant, known as *san qi hua*, is used for high blood pressure, dizziness, vertigo, and hypertensive tinnitus.

Other Herbs in This Category
Human hair (burnt): *xue yu tan, Crinis carbonisatus*
Mugwort leaf: *ai ye, Artemesia folium*
Burnet-bloodwort root: *di yu, Sanguisorba radix*
Lotus receptacle: *lian fang, Receptaculum nelumbinis nuciferae*

Herbs that Warm the Interior

Herbs in this group treat interior cold patterns that may have originated in the interior or have invaded from the exterior. The symptoms of interior cold include feeling chilled, having cold hands or feet, a pale complexion, slow pulse, loose stool, a preference for warm liquids, and a slow metabolism. herbs that warm the interior are often used in conjunction with herbs that tonify the yang to increase or speed up metabolism.

Rou Gui   (Cinnamon bark, *Cortex cinnamomi cassiae*)

Properties of Chinese Medicine   Acrid and sweet taste, hot temperature

Clinical Functions   *Rou gui* warms the kidneys and the center, fortifies the yang, warms the channels, promotes menstruation, and leads fire back to its source

Part of Plant Used   Bark

Cautions and Contraindications   *Rou gui* is contraindicated for kidney yin deficiency heat patterns. Use cautiously during pregnancy.

Daily Dosage and Administration   *Rou gui* should not be cooked, but rather ground to powder or used in pills (three-tenths to three grams)

Notes   Cinnamon bark is used for deficiency yang patterns that manifest as impotence, premature ejaculation, menstrual pain, cold or weak back or legs, or lower back pain. It is also used in kidney deficient asthma formulas where the lungs cannot grasp the Qi (see Asthma in

Chapter 6, "Treatment of Ailments From A to Z").

Rou gui is used in small amounts to return fire to its source. In these cases, the weak yang has floated upward and created symptoms such as flushed face, wheezing, and severe sweating, together with weak or cold lower extremities. This pattern is called Waning Fire at the Gate of Vitality and is characterized by simultaneous hot or inflammatory conditions in the upper body and cold or deficient symptoms in the lower body.

Other Herbs in This Category
Dried ginger: *gan jiang, Rhizoma zingeberis officinalis*
Evodia fruit: *wu zhu yu, Fructus evodiae rutaecarpa*
Pepper: *chuan jiao, Fructus zanthoxyli bungeani*
Cloves: *ding xiang, Flos caryophylli*

Herbs That Strengthen (Tonifying Herbs)

These herbs supplement body processes, substances, or structures that have been weakened or depleted. These herbs are also used to promote physiologic normalcy (righteous Qi) when abnormal conditions (illness) persist, allowing the body's normal processes and defenses to defeat the pathogenic influences (evil Qi). They are most often used in deficient or chronic conditions, but are also used in small amounts, long-term, to optimize heath. As a general rule, when the illness comes from the exterior, such as in the case of cold or flu, tonics are suspended. They are resumed only after the illness has been expelled, because taking tonics during cold or flu can prolong or deepen the disease.

Herbs That Tonify the Qi

Huang Qi   (Milk-vetch root, *Radix astragali*)

Properties of Chinese Medicine   Sweet taste, slightly warm temperature

Clinical Functions   *Huang qi* tonifies the spleen, benefits the Qi, raises the Qi of the spleen and stomach, stabilizes the exterior, and promotes healing, urination, and the discharge of pus

Part of Plant Used   Root

Cautions and Contraindications   *Huang qi* is contraindicated for people with heat signs caused by deficient yin (unless modified by other herbs), and is contraindicated during cold or flu (unless modified by other herbs)

Daily Dosage and Administration   Boiled: nine to thirty grams; powdered: two to six grams

Notes   In the *Essentials of the Materia Medica* (1694 AD), *huang qi* (*Astragalus*) was called "the senior of all herbs." It tonifies the spleen, stomach, Qi, and blood, and benefits the *wei Qi* (immune system). Research has shown *huang qi* to lower blood pressure and increase endurance. This herb, recognized for its action to increase the body's resistance, is now considered one of the world's greatest immune tonics.

Astragalus root has many different functions. The following combinations illustrate this point:

- *Astragalus* + ginseng (*ren shen*): benefits the Qi and enhances immunity, particularly when weak Qi results in shortness of breath, fatigue, and low appetite.
- *Astragalus* + cicumfuaga (*sheng ma*) and/or bupleurum (*chai hu*): for prolapse (falling down) of the organs due to weakening of the Qi's lifting quality. Examples of prolapse are hernia, hemorrhoids, varicose veins, and uterine and anal prolapse.
- *Astragalus* (*huang qi*) + *Ledebouriella* (*fang feng*): for spontaneous or excessive sweating due to weak protective Qi.
- *Astragalus* (*huang qi*) + *Stephania* (*fang ji*): for edema in the upper body.
- *Astragalus* (*huang qi*) + cinnamon branches (*gui zhi*): for pain and/or numbness due to low Qi.
- *Astragalus* (*huang qi*) + oyster shell (*mu li*): for night sweats caused by deficient yin and Qi.
- *Astragalus* (*huang qi*) + dioscorea (*shan yao*): for diabetes.

Ren Shen   (Ginseng, *Radix panax ginseng*)

Properties of Chinese Medicine   Sweet and slightly bitter taste, slightly warm temperature

Clinical Functions *Ren shen* tonifies the original Qi, lungs, and spleen, benefits the yin by generating fluids, and calms the spirit

Part of Plant Use Root

Cautions and Contraindications Ren shen is contraindicated with heat signs of any origin (unless modified by other herbs) and with high blood pressure. Overdose or overuse can cause headache, hypertension, or insomnia. Traditionally, ginseng was considered antagonistic, and not to be taken together with *wu ling zhi* (flying squirrel feces).

Daily Dosage and Administration Good ginseng is expensive. To maximize the extraction of its valuable components, ginseng root should be sliced into dime-sized pieces before boiling. To slice rock-hard roots, microwave them first for about four seconds. This softens the root instantly. Ginseng is often boiled alone in a double boiler. Use a low boil or simmer for about one hour.

Boiled The general dose is three to nine grams. To calm the spirit, use one to three grams or less. In cases of shock due to blood loss, thirty to fifty grams can be given. Double boiling is preferred. Slow boil herb slices for about one hour, and drink the tea on an empty stomach.

Powdered or in Pill Form Use one half to two grams. To calm the spirit use one to three tenths of a gram.

Eaten Raw Ginseng slices can be sucked, chewed, and swallowed. Ginseng will slice easily after it has been warmed in the oven for a few minutes or in the microwave for a few seconds.

Notes When people refer to ginseng, they generally mean Oriental ginseng, also known as panax ginseng. Ginseng is a perennial plant of the *Araliaceae* family. It grows on the slopes of ravines and in shady mountain forests. It bears five leaves on a single stalk at maturity. A gray flower blooms in spring and later turns into a cluster of dark red fruit. It grows to between seven and twenty-one inches in height. The root is creamy yellow or white, sometimes taking the shape of a human body. The more it resembles a human body, the more it is prized.

The taste of panax ginseng is sweet and bitter. When untreated, its nature is slightly warming. When steamed with *fu zi* (aconite), it becomes warmer and thus more stimulating. As a tonic, it is used to increase strength, increase blood volume, promote life and appetite—and, taken in small amounts, it also calms the spirit. It is used alone or in formulas for general weakness, deficient Qi patterns, and for recovery after illness or blood loss. Ginseng is one of the principal herbs in the famous spleen tonic Four Gentlemen (see chapter 5, "Famous Herbal Medicines"). Panax ginseng is the single herb known to strengthen the "original Qi" (*yuan qi*) and thus prolong life. This accounts for its great value and popularity.

The Price of Ginseng   The price of ginseng (Oriental or American) can vary greatly. Soup-grade ginseng roots can sell for a few dollars at the grocery, while the highest grades will bring over $10,000 per root. Ginseng roots gathered from the wild are far more costly than those cultivated on a farm. Wild-crafted roots will also not contain traces of the fungicides that are used on cultivated roots.

Roots that resemble a human form are more valuable. Big roots are better than small ones. Thick roots are preferable to thin. Old roots are more prized than fresh ones. Strong characteristic taste and smell also indicate the strength and price of ginseng roots. Buyer beware: Siberian ginseng root (*ci wu jia*) is often marketed as ginseng. but it is nothing at all like ginseng. Siberian ginseng is cheap, and should cost only a fraction of the price of Oriental or American ginseng (see profile in this chapter under Herbs to Expel Dampness).

Ginseng Extracts (Pills and Liquids)   Ginseng (like any herb) is made up of hundreds of different chemicals. Standardized ginseng extracts are rated by the percentage of ginsanocides they contain. Scientists believe these chemicals create ginseng's effects. Marketers believe that consumers favor standardization. Herbalists, however, believe that the effects of any herb depend on the interaction of its many chemical components. That is why most herbologists prefer whole herbs or simple water extractions to standardized extracts, which are usually taken from inferior herbs that cannot be sold whole due to poor appearance, taste, or potency. Low-temperature water extracts, which have not been chemically manipulated to standardize ginsanocides, are more like the herb as it is found in nature. These extracts are, of course, only as potent as the herbs from which they came.

Preparation of Ginseng Panax ginseng is usually steamed with aconite or other herbs to enhance its strength. This is called red ginseng. It has a warm nature. Also available is white ginseng, which is unprocessed panax ginseng. Milder white ginseng is more appropriate when the user has too much heat. Its cooler nature is less stimulating and does not aggravate hot or inflammatory conditions.

Organic Ginseng Ginseng that is truly gathered in the wild (wildcrafted) is likely free of fertilizers and pesticides. However, to be called "organic," ginseng must be certified by a third party organization recognized under the Organic Food Production Act (OFPA). This law can be accessed online. Methods of certification vary from state to state, and, until very recently, there were no Chinese certification agencies recognized by federal authorities. This picture is beginning to change, and markets are adapting to the demand for organic products.

Ling Chih (*ling zi* [Chinese], or Rei Shi or Reishi [Japanese] Mushroom, *Ganoderma lucida*

Properties of Chinese Medicine Sweet taste, neutral temperature

Clinical Functions *Ling chih* tonifies Qi and calms the spirit

Part of Plant Used Fruiting body

Cautions and Contraindications None noted

Daily Dosage and Administration Boiled: three to thirty grams; powdered: one-half to six grams

Notes The most famous tonic mushroom of China, *Ling chih*, means spiritual mushroom. It benefits heart Qi, tonifies the middle burner (liver, stomach, spleen), and is said to increase insight and intelligence. It is used traditionally as a Qi tonic and sedative, and is considered an important immune-enhancing and anti-stress herb. *Ling chih* is used in many anti-cancer and radiation-relieving formulas.

Other Herbs in This Category

Poor man's ginseng: *dang shen*
Yam root: *shan yao, Dioscorea opposista radix*

Licorice root: *gan cao, Glycyrrhiza uralensis radix*
Atractylodes rhizome: *bai zhu, Rhizoma Atractylodes*
Jujube fruit: *da zao, Fructus ziziphi jujubae*
Barley malt sugar: *yi tang, Saccharum granorum*

Herbs That Tonify the Yang

As the kidney is the root of the body's yang, most of these herbs also tonify the kidney. As the yang is the root of activity, deficiencies of yang produce symptoms of low activity. The herbs in this category treat exhaustion, feeling cold, weak lower back and lower extremities, impotence, premature ejaculation, bed wetting, frequent urination, watery vaginal discharge, wheezing, and cock's crow diarrhea (diarrhea at daybreak). In modern terms, these herbs are thought to help regulate metabolism, promote growth, strengthen sexual function, and increase resistance.

Dong Chong Xia Cao   (Cordyceps, *Cordyceps sinensis*)

Properties of Chinese Medicine   Sweet taste, neutral temperature

Clinical Functions   Dong chong xia cao nourishes the lungs and fortifies the kidneys

Part of Plant Used   Whole fungus, including the insect larva from which it grows

Cautions and Contraindications   Do not use during cold or flu.

Daily Dosage and Administration   Boiled: three to twelve grams; powdered: one-half to two grams

Notes   Restorative and tonifying *dong chong xia cao* nourishes the lungs and *lung yin* fortifies the kidneys, and builds Qi. Because it tonifies both the yin and yang and is a very safe substance, it can be taken over a long period of time. *Dong chong xia cao* improves lung function and has been traditionally used for wheezing, chronic cough, and fatigue, as well as the effects of chemotherapiy and radiation. It boosts the immune system's resistance to disease and has even been used by Chinese athletes to enhance performance.

Cordyceps is one of the most valued traditional Chinese herbs. It consists of the dried fungus that grows on caterpillar larvae. For medication, the fruiting body (fungus) and the worm (caterpillar) are used together.

In one study, the water extracts from cordyceps were analyzed for their content of nucleosides and polysaccharides; the results showed that the worm had a chemical composition similar to the fruiting body. In addition, both the fruiting body and worm of cordyceps showed similar potency in their antioxidant activities. These results suggest that the function of the worm in cordyceps is to provide a growth medium for the fruiting body.

Yin Yang Huo (Horny goat weed, *Epimedium sagittatum*)

Properties of Chinese Medicine Acrid, sweet taste, warm temperature

Clinical Functions Yin yang huo tonifies the kidneys, fortifies the yang, and expels wind cold dampness from the joints of the lower extremities

Part of Plant Used Aerial parts

Cautions and Contraindications Yin yang huo is contraindicated in yin deficiency heat conditions, and is contraindicated in cases of excessive sexual drive or wet dreams. Not for prolonged use, it can damage the yin fluids.

Daily Dosage and Administration Boiled: three to twelve grams; powdered: one-half to three grams. Note: *yin yang huo* should not be ingested as a tea over long periods of time.

Notes Yin yang huo is a legendary sex tonic. It tonifies the kidneys, fortifies the yin and yang, and expels wind cold dampness (good for joint pain). Research has shown that it increases sexual activity, increases sperm production, stimulates the sensory nerves, and increases sexual desire. Use it together with *gou qi zi* (goji berries) and/or *wu wei zi* (*schizandra*) to enhance its sexual effects or for treating impotence or infertility.

Other Herbs in This Category
Gecko lizard: *ge jie, Gekko gecko Linneaus*
Fenugreek seed: *hu lu ba, Semen trigonellae foeni-graeci*
Walnut meat: *hu tao ren, Semen juglandis regiae*

Golden eye grass: *xian mao, Rhizoma curculinginis orchioidis*
Temperate rubber tree bark: *du zhong, Cortex eucommia ulmoidis*
Dodder seeds: *tu su zi, Semen cuscutae*
Human placenta: *zi he che, Placenta hominis*
Pipe fish: *hai long, Colenognathus hardwickii*
Sea horse: *hai ma: hippocampus*

Herbs That Tonify the Yin

Herbs from this category nourish and moisten the lungs, stomach, liver, kidneys, or intestines.

Xi Yang Shen   (American ginseng, *Radix panacis quinquefolii*)

Properties of Chinese Medicine   Sweet, slightly bitter taste, cool temperature

Clinical Functions   *Xi yang shen* benefits the Qi and yin of the lung, stomach, and kidney, and generates fluids

Part of Plant Used   Root

Cautions and Contraindications   *Xi yang shen* is contraindicated for cold or damp stomach patterns.

Daily Dosage and Administration   Boiled: three to nine grams; powdered, one-half to two grams

Notes   American ginseng (*xi yang shen*) is very different from Oriental ginseng (*ren shen*). Oriental ginseng builds Qi energy; American ginseng builds yin fluids. Prized almost as much as Oriental ginseng, it can be used for any yin deficiency, with or without heat signs. It treats weakness, dryness, irritability, and thirst of yin deficiencies and of fevers, or in the aftermath of fevers. Combine it with *shi gao* (gypsum) and/or *zhi mu* (Anemarrhena) to heighten this effect. Though it grows wild in many areas of the United States, the best quality is said to come from Wisconsin.

Other Herbs in This Category

Chinese asparagus tuber: *tian men dong, Tuber asparagi cochinchinensis*
Lily bulb: *bai he, Bulbus lilii*

Privet fruit: *nu zhen zi, Fructus ligustri lucidi*
Land tortoise shell: *gui ban, Plastrum testudunis*
White fungus: *bai mu er, Fructificatio tremellae*
Sesame seeds: *hei zhi ma, Semen sesami indici*

Herbs That Astringe

These herbs help to contain things, usually fluids like urine or sweat. They may also be used to contain stool, Qi, or *jing* (essence). They treat leakages, such as frequent urination, excessive sweating, and chronic and acute diarrhea. Some are useful in certain bleeding conditions. Often, astringents are combined with tonifying herbs to prevent the leakage of Qi, blood, essence, and the like, while these substances are being restored.

Wu Wei Zi (Schisandra fruit, *Fructus schisandrae chinensis*)

Properties of Chinese Medicine Sour taste, warm temperature

Clinical Functions *Wu wei zi* contains the leakage of lung Qi and kidney essence, stops diarrhea, restrains excessive sweating, and calms the spirit

Part of Plant Used Fruit

Cautions and Contraindications Do not take *wu wei zi* with cold, flu, or fever. It is used for chronic coughs, not used for the early stages of new coughs. Use this herb cautiously when you tend to be constipated. Note: a thin white crust that may be found on the berries does not affect their quality.

Daily Dosage and Administration Boiled: three to nine grams to relieve symptoms, one-half to six grams for maintenance. Powdered: one-half to two grams. Medicinal wine: soak fifty-six grams, or about two ounces, of *wu wei zi* (schisandra) in one liter of rice wine or other drinkable alcohol. Use a glass container, and allow it to stand in a cool dry place, away from direct sunlight, for at least a week (longer is better). You can add more of your favorite tonic herbs. Stir daily. Drink one ounce daily as a general tonic.

Notes *Wu wei zi*, shizandra, is an amazing, very versatile and safe herb. *Wu* (five) *wei* (flavor) *zi* (fruit) has five main functions. It reduces the leakage of lung Qi to stop coughing and wheezing. It rejuvenates kidney energy to reduce urinary frequency, stops diarrhea, and astringes excessive sweating. And it calms the spirit to aid in the treatment of insomnia. It is thought to do all this through its ability to astringe *jing* (essence) and prevent the leakage of essential Qi and fluids. *Wu wei zi* is rarely used alone. Its actions are more powerful in the following five combinations:

Wu wei zi + *shan yao* (yam root): for cough and wheezing
Wu wei zi + *gou qi zi* (goji berries): for frequent urination
Wu wei zi + *bu gu zi* (Psoralea): for chronic diarrhea
Wu wei zi + *huang qi* (Astragalus): for excessive sweating
Wu wei zi + *suan zao ren* (sour date seed): for insomnia

Other Herbs in This Category
Nutmeg: *rou dou kou, Semen myristicae*
Pomegranate husk: *shi li pi, Pericarpium punicae granati*
Lotus seed: *lian zi, Semen nelumbinis nuciferae*
Chinese raspberry: *fu pen zi, Fructus rubi*
Ginkgo nut: *yin guo, Semen ginkgo bilobae*
Wheat: *fu xiao mai, Semen tritici aestivi levis*
Cuttle-fish bone: *hai piao xiao, Os sepiae*
Egg case of the praying mantis: *sang piao xiao, Ootheca mantidis*

Herbs That Nourish the Heart and Settle the Spirit

This category is divided into two subcategories, Herbs that Nourish the Heart and Herbs that Settle the Spirit. Herbs that nourish the heart generally supplement the yin of the heart or the heart blood. A well-nourished heart makes a comfortable home for the spirit (*shen*), which resides in the heart.

Herbs that settle or calm the spirit—mostly shells, stones, and minerals—are usually heavy substances, and have a sedating effect. They are thought to weigh on the heart to settle an anxious spirit. Some of these substances contain heavy metals and should not be taken by children or over long periods of time.

Herbs That Nourish the Heart

Suan Zao Ren (Sour jujube seed, *Ziziphi semen*)

Properties of Chinese Medicine Sweet, sour taste, neutral temperature

Clinical Functions *Suan zao ren* nourishes the yin of the heart and liver, restrains sweating, and lubricates the stool.

Part of Plant Used Seed

Cautions and Contraindications People with diarrhea should use *suan zao ren* cautiously

Daily Dosage and Administration Crush seeds before boiling. Boiled: nine to eighteen grams; powdered: one to four grams.

Notes *Suan zao ren* is the seed of *da zao* (Chinese sour date fruit) which is classified as a tonify Qi herb. Used for heart palpitations, insomnia, and agitation, *suan zao ren* nourishes the heart. The seed has much stronger insomnia-relieving properties than the fruit, but the fruit is a better blood tonic. People who suffer from blood-deficient insomnia can use both together. The seeds have the additional property of lubricating the intestines, so be careful using this if you tend to have loose stool or diarrhea.

Herbs That Settle the Spirit

Mu Li (Oyster shell, *Concha ostrea*)

Long Gu (Dragon bone, *Os draconic* [fossilized bone])

Properties of Chinese Medicine *Mu li*: salty and astringent taste, cool temperature; long gu: sweet and astringent taste, neutral temperature

Clinical Functions Both *mu li* and *long gu* settle and calm the spirit; both calm the liver and restrain rising yang. Both prevent the leakage of fluids. *Mu li* (oyster shell) also absorbs acidity, and softens hardness. *Long gu* (fossilized bone) is used topically for sores that resist healing.

Part of Plant Used Shell (*mu li)*, fossilized bone (*long gu*)

Cautions and Contraindications Because of their astringency, neither of these herbs should be used during an exterior disease such as cold or flu, where the exterior must be kept open in order to expel the invading pathogen. Oyster shell is also considered to react adversely when combined with *ma huang* (Ephedra), *wu zhu yu* (Evodia), or *xi xin* (Herba asari). Long-term use of mineral herbs is discouraged because of the possibility of heavy metal accumulation in the body.

Daily Dosage and Administration *Long gu* (fossil bone): fifteen to fifty grams; *mu li* (oyster shell): nine to fifty grams. Both require extra cooking time and should be pre-boiled for twenty or thirty minutes before adding other herbs.

Notes These two mineral-rich substances are categorized as herbs that settle the spirit. Most herbs in this group are minerals or shells, heavy substances said to anchor the Spirit (*shen*) to the heart. Settling herbs also weigh down rebellious and uprising liver Qi to relieve the related symptoms of headache, dizziness, flushed face, or an angry or cantankerous disposition. These mineral herbs also suppress vomiting, belching, and hiccups, all signs of rebellious stomach Qi.

These two herbs in particular, oyster shell and fossil bone, have additional astringent properties that help in the containment of fluids and find use in the treatment of night sweats, nocturnal emissions, and premature ejaculation. Oyster shell has the additional property of softening the hard and is used in many formulas aimed at dissipating nodules, goiters, and other lumps in the neck.

Other Herbs in This Category
Lodestone: *ci shi, Magnetitum*
Pearl: *zhen zhu, Magarita*
Amber: *hu po, Succinum*
Cinnabar: *zhu sha, Cinnabaris*

Aromatic Herbs That Open the Orifices

These substances are primarily used for locked-up or closed syndrome (*bi zheng*) that can manifest as hot closed syndrome with symptoms of fainting, coma, stroke, locked jaw, clenched fists, and spastic paralysis. Or it can be cold closed syndrome, presenting with sudden collapse, pallor, cold body, and a slow pulse.

Bing Pian   (Borneol camphor, *Dryobalanops aromatica*)

Properties of Chinese Medicine   Acrid and bitter taste, cool temperature

Clinical Functions   *Bing pian* opens the orifices, revives the senses, clears heat, relieves pain, and dissipates nodules

Part of Plant Used   Sap

Cautions and Contraindications   Do not apply *bing pian* over the abdomen during pregnancy

Daily Dosage and Administration   Do not boil. Powdered: small dosages recommended, one-tenth to one-third gram. Use only in pills and powders.

Notes   You may recognize *bing pian*, Borneol camphor, as smelling salts. It is the highly aromatic processed resin of the camphor tree. According to Chinese theory, *bing pian* opens the orifices and revives the senses. Sniff it alone or together with musk (*she xiang*) for fainting and convulsions. Use it together with borax (*peng sha*) topically for pain, swelling and suppuration (discharge of pus) of the eye, ear, nose, and throat.

Other Herbs in Category
   Musk: *she xiang, Moschus moschiferi secretio*
   Sweet flag: *chang pu, Acori graminei rhizoma*
   Cattle gallstone: *niu huang, Bovis calculus*

Herbs to Extinguish Interior Wind and Stop Tremors

The movement of interior wind is characterized by headaches, dizziness, blurred vision, ear ringing (tinnitus), hypertension, palpitations, spasms, and stroke. This is often the result of distress in the liver and kidneys. However, it may also arise out of deficient blood or as a result of high fevers or sudden loss of fluid. Substances from this category are used together with herbs to transform phlegm to treat and prevent these conditions. These herbs appear to have the effects of antihypertensive drugs or mild sedatives.

Gou Teng   (Gambir vine, *Ramulus uncaria cum uncis*)

Properties of Chinese Medicine   Sweet taste, cool temperature

Clinical Functions   *Gou teng* extinguishes wind, clears heat, and pacifies the liver

Part of Plant Used   Stems and thorns

Cautions and Contraindications   None

Daily Dosage and Administration   Boiled: use three to nine grams. *Gou teng* should not be cooked longer than ten minutes. Powdered: use one-half to two grams.

Tian Ma   (Gastrodia rhizome, *Rhizoma gastrodia elatae*)

Properties of Chinese Medicine   Sweet taste, slightly warm temperature

Clinical Functions   *Tian ma* extinguishes wind, pacifies the liver, and disperses painful obstructions.

Part of Plant Used   Rhizome

Cautions and Contraindications   None

Daily Dosage and Administration   Boiled: three to nine grams; powdered: one-half to two grams.

Notes   A dynamic duo, *gou teng* and *tian ma* are often packaged together. *Gou teng* extinguishes wind and relieves spasms. It has a cooling nature and is always included when heat underlies the interior wind, a frequent occurrence since wind moves and heat makes things move. *Tian ma* is used for problems that arise either from heat or from deficient blood. It is used for many kinds of headaches, including migraines, and for strokes resulting in paralysis and numbness in the extremities.

Other Herbs in This Category

Abalone shell: *shi jue ming, Concha haliotidis*
Earthworm: *di long, Lumbricus*
Scorpion: *quan xie, Buthus martensi*
Centipede: *wu gong, Scolopendra subsinipes*
Silkworm: *jiang can, Bombyx batryticatus*

Herbs that Expel Parasites

If you have traveled in China, you know that hygienic conditions in many areas fall short of Western standards. The general rule is "don't drink the water." The Chinese people have considerable experience dealing with parasites and pestilence caused by lax hygiene. Most of the herbs in this category treat intestinal parasites. They are neither as strong as nor as fast acting as anti-parasitic chemicals. However, they are ultimately lethal to these organisms. To their benefit, these herbs are far less toxic to humans than pharmaceuticals, and many believe their action is longer lasting. They can also be combined with spleen tonics to help repair the damage to the digestion inflicted by the invading parasites.

Bing Lang (Betel nut, *Quisqualis indica fructus*)

Properties of Chinese Medicine Acrid, bitter taste, warm temperature

Clinical Functions *Bing lang*, betel nut, kills parasites, including tapeworm, fasciolopsis, pinworms, roundworms, and blood flukes. Drains Qi, blood, and food downward, and promotes urination.

Part of Plant Used Seed

Cautions and Contraindications Use *bing lang* with caution with loose stool. In Asia, many people chew the bitter-tasting betel nut daily. It produces a mild narcotic effect, and when chewed over time, the nut colors the user's mouth red. However, habitual use causes gum disease, hunger pangs, and diarrhea, and deadens the taste buds. Overdoses may cause increased salivation, vomiting, and stupor.

Daily Dosage and Administration Boiled when blended with other herbs: six to twelve grams. Boiled alone for tapeworm: thirty to two hundred grams. Powdered when blended with other herbs: one to three grams. Powdered when used alone: one to six grams.

Notes *Bing lang* is especially effective in killing tapeworms. Use it together with *wu mei* (sour plum) and *gan cao* (licorice root) for fasciolopsiasis. Combine it with *nan gua zi* (pumpkin seeds) to dislodge and expel tapeworms. The downward-draining property of this herb also helps expel parasites from the body.

Other Herbs in This Category

Pumpkin seeds: *nan gua zi, Cucurbita moschata semen*
Garlic bulb: *da suan, Alli sativi bulbus*
Paste of stinking elm fruit: *wu yi, Pasta ulmi macrocarpi*

Herbs for Topical Application

Herbs in this category treat topical and usually localized conditions such as bleeding, inflammation, infection, swelling, pain, and the healing of cuts, sores, and lesions. They can be administered as powders, plasters, ointments, washes, steams, fumigants, and soaks.

Liu Huang (Sulphur)

Properties of Chinese Medicine   Sour, hot taste, poisonous

Clinical Functions   Sulpher detoxifies poison and kills parasites; taken internally, it strengthens the yang

Part of Plant Used   Mineral element

Cautions and Contraindications   *Lui huang*, sulphur, is forbidden during pregnancy, and is contraindicated for people who exhibit heat signs from deficient yin. Use caution when taken internally.

Daily Dosage and Administration   Apply any quantity topically. Not used in boiled decoctions. Powdered for internal use: one-half to six grams.

Notes   Sulphur (*liu huang*) has been used in Chinese medicine since before 200 BC in topical applications to cure scabies, ringworm, and skin infections. However, sulfa drugs (sulphur-based antibiotics) weren't discovered in the West until over 2,000 years later. Good news travels slowly. This herb is considered poisonous, but can be taken internally in small amounts to tonify fire in the gate of vitality. This is a deficiency marked by low sex drive, weak lower back and knees, and a sensation of cold in the body.

Other Herbs in This Category

Hornet's nest: *lu feng fang*
Alum: *ming fan*, aluminum and potasium
Borax: *peng sha, sodium tetraborate*
Camphor: *zhang nao, d-camphora*

Appendix 1

Chinese Herb List and Pronunciation Guide

How to Pronounce Chinese Words

It's hard for Westerners to pronounce Chinese words. Aside from the fact that Chinese uses a tonal system that radically changes the meaning of a word, the Chinese language also includes several sounds not found at all in English.

Pinyin is a system that uses the Latin alphabet to represent sounds in Mandarin Chinese. The sounds represented in pinyin by the letters b and g correspond more to the sounds we know as p and k. The letters j, q, x, or zh designate sounds that aren't found in English at all. Westerners attempting to speak words containing these letters are usually met with blank expressions.

Pinyin	Sounds Like
b	unaspirated p, as in spit
p	aspirated p, as in pit
m	same as English

f	same as in English
d	unaspirated t, as in stop
t	aspirated t, as in top
n	same as in English
l	something between the l in English and the continental r
g	unaspirated k, as in skill
k	aspirated k, as in kill
h	same as English h when followed by an a
j	like q, but unaspirated
q	like the ch in church
x	like sh, but take the sound and pass it backwards along the tongue until it is clear of the tongue tip; very similar to the final sound in the German word, *ich*
zh	ch with no aspiration; very similar to the word merger in American English, but not voiced
ch	as in chin, but with the tongue curled upwards; very similar to nurture or tree in American English, but strongly aspirated
sh	as in shinbone, but with the tongue curled upwards; very similar to undershirt in American English
r	similar to the English r in rank
z	unaspirated c (halfway between beds and bets, like the word suds)
c	like ts, aspirated (more common example is cats)
s	as in sun
w	may be considered as an initial or a final, and may be pronounced as w or u as in English
y	may be considered as an initial or a final, and may be pronounced as y or i as in English

List of Chinese Herbs

There are over ten thousand medicinal substances listed in all the Chinese medical pharmacopoeias, so the following list is obviously not comprehensive. Herbs are listed by Latin names because they are listed that way on medicine bottles. Latin names are also more consistently applied and spelled than pinyin names, even if they are no easier to pronounce. Note that italicized English names are the literal translations of Chinese names and are used when common English names are unknown.

Latin Name	Pinyin	English Name or Literal Translation	Category
Acanthopanax gracilistylus	*wu jia pi*	siberian ginseng root bark	dispels wind, damp
Achyranthes bidentata	*(huai) niu xi*	ox knee	vitalizes blood
Aconitum carmichaeli	*fu zi*	aconite	warms interior, expels cold
Acorus gramineus	*shi chang pi*	acorus	aromatic, opens orifices
Adenophora stricta	*sha shen*	sand root	tonifies yin
Agastache rugosa	*huo xiang*	patchouli	transforms damp
Agrimonia pilosa	*xian he cao*	agrimony	stops bleeding
Alianthus	*chun pi*	tree of heaven bark	astringent
Akebia quinata	*mu tong*	wood with holes	drains damp
Albizzia julibrissin	*he huan pi*	mimosa tree	nourishes heart, calms spirit
Allium sativum	*da suan*	garlic	expels parasites
Allium tuberosum	*jiu zi*	chives	tonifies yang
Aloes herba	*lu hui*	aloe	purgative
Anemarrhena	*zhi mu*	know mother	clears heat, drains fire

Angelica dahurica	*bai zhi*	angelica root	releases exterior, warms
Angelica pubescens	*du huo*	self-reliant	dispels wind, damp
Angelica sinenses	*dang gui*	tang kwei	tonifies blood
Arctium lappa	*niu bang zi*	burdock	releases exterior, cools
Arecae catechu	*bing lang*	betel nut	kills parasites
Arisaema consanguineum	*tian nan xing*	jack-in-the-pulpit	transforms cold phlegm
Artemisia annua	*qing hao*	sweet annie	relieves summer heat
Artemisia vulgaris	*ai ye*	mugwort leaf	stops bleeding
Asparagus cochinchinensis	*tian dong*	asparagus tuber	tonifies yin
Aster tataricus	*zi wan*	aster root	relieves coughing, wheezing
Astragalus chinensis	*sha yuan ji li*	Astragalus seed	tonifies yang
Astragalus membranaceus	*huang qi*	Astragalus root	tonifies *qi*
Atractylodes alba	*bai zhu*	Atractylodes root	tonifies *qi*
Belamcanda chinensis	*she gan*	blackberry lily	clears heat, cleans toxins
Benicasa hispida	*donggua ren*	winter melon seed	drains damp
Biota orientalis	*ce bai ye*	arborvitae leaf	stops bleeding
Biota orientalis	*bai zi ren*	arborvitae seed	nourishes heart, calms spirit
Bletilla striata	*bai ji*	bletilla rhizome	stops bleeding
Borneol	*bing pien*	Borneol camphor	opens orifices
Brassica alba	*bai jie zi*	mustard seed	transforms cold phlegm

Brucae javanica	*ya dan zi*	crow gallbladder seed	clears heat, cleans toxins
Bupleurum chinense	*chai hu*	hare's ear root	releases exterior, cools
Canabis sativa	*huo ma ren*	marijuana seeds	lubricating purgative
Carthami flos	*hong hua*	safflower	vitalizes blood
Celosia argentea	*qing xiang zi*	celosia seed	clears heat, drains fire
Chaenomeles speciosa	*mu gua*	flow quince	dispels wind and damp
Chrysanthemum	*ju hua*	chrysanthemum	releases exterior, cools
Cimicifuga dahurica	*sheng ma*	black cohosh	releases exterior, cools
Cirsium japonicum	*da ji*	pink beauty	stops bleeding
Citrullus vulgaris	*xi gua*	watermelon	relieves summer heat
Clematis hexapetala	*wei ling xian*	clematis root	dispels wind and damp
Cnidium monnieri	*shechuangzi*	snake bed seeds	external application
Codonopsis pilosula	*dang shen*	relative root	tonifies *qi*
Coix lachryma jobi	*yi yi ren*	Job's tears	drains damp
Coptis chinensis	*huang lian*	golden thread	clears heat, dries damp
Cornus officinalis	*shan zhu yu*	cornelian cherry	astringent
Corydalis yanhusuo	*yan hu suo*	corydalis	vitalizes blood
Crataegus pinnatifida	*shan zha*	hawthorn berry	relieve food stagnation
Cucurbita moschata	*nan gua zi*	pumpkin seeds	expels parasites

Curcuma longa	*yu jin*	turmeric tuber	vitalizes blood
Curcuma longa	*jiang huang*	turmeric rhizome	vitalizes blood
Cyperus rotundus	*xiang fu*	nut-grass rhizome	regulates Qi
Daucus carota	*he shi*	carrot seed	expels parasites
Dianthus chinensis	*qu mai*	china pink	drains damp
Dictamnus dasycarpus	*bai xian pi*	gas plant	clears heat, cleans toxins
Dioscorea opposita	*shan yao*	Chinese yam root	tonifies Qi
Dioscorea tokoro	*bei xie*	yam rhizome	drains damp
Dipsacus asper	*xu duan*	teasel root	tonifies yang
Dolichos lablab	*bian dou*	hyacinth bean	relieves summer heat
Eclipta prostrata	*han lian cao*	false daisy	tonifies yin
Elsholzia ciliata	*xiang ru*	aromatic madder	releases exterior, warms
Ephedra sinica	*ma huang*	Ephedra	releases exterior, warms
Ephedra sinica	*mahuanggen*	Ephedra root	astringent
Equisetum hiemale	*mu zei*	horsetail	releases exterior, cools
Eucommia ulmoides	*du zhong*	rubber tree bark	tonifies yang
Eupatorium fortunei	*pei lan*	ornamental orchid	transforms damp
Euphorbia pekinensis	*da ji*	spurge root	draining, harsh expellants
Foeniculum vulgare	*xiaohui xiang*	fennel	warms interior, expel cold
Forsythia suspensa	*lian qiao*	forsythia	clears heat, cleans toxins
Fraxinus bungeana	*qin pi*	korean ash bark	clears heat, dries damp

Gentiana macrophylla	*qin jiao*	gentian root	dispels wind and damp
Gentiana Scabrae	*long dan cao*	dragon gallbladder herb	clears heat, dries damp
Ginkgo biloba	*bia guo*	gingko seed	astringent
Gleditsia sinensis	*zao jiao*	honeylocust fruit	relieves coughing, wheezing
Glycine max	*dou juan*	fermented soybean	relieves summer heat
Glycyrrhiza uralensis	*gan cao*	licorice root	tonifies Qi
Heraclelum lanatum	*du huo*	cow parsnip root	dispels wind and damp
Hordeum vulgare	*mai ya*	barley sprout	relieves food stagnation
Houttuynia cordata	*yu xing cao*	fish smell herb	clears heat, cleans toxins
Inula japonica	*xuan fu hua*	upturned flower	transforms cold phlegm
Isatis tinctoria	*da qing ye*	woad leaf	clears heat, cleans toxin
Isatis tinctoria	*ban lan gen*	woad root	clears heat, cleans toxins
Kochia scoparia	*di fu zi*	summer cypress	drains damp
Leonurus heterophyllus	*yi mu cao*	Chinese mother-wort	vitalizes blood
Ligusticum chuanxiong	*chuan xiong*	Sezhuan lovage	vitalizes blood
Ligusticum jeholense	*gao ben*	Chinese lovage	releases exterior, warms
Ligustrum lucidum `	*nu zhen zi*	shining privet seed	tonifies yin
Lilium longiflorum	*bai he*	lily bulb	tonifies yin

Lindera strychnifolia	wu yao	Lindera root	regulates Qi
Lithospermum	zi cao	groomwell root	clears heat, cools blood
Lonicera japonica	jin yin hua	honeysuckle	clears heat, cleans toxin
Lophatherum gracile	dan zhu ye	bland bamboo leaf	clears heat, drains fire
Luffa acutangula	si gua luo	luffa	vitalizes blood
Lycium chinense	di gu pi	matrimony vine	clears heat, cools blood
Lycium chinense	gou qi zi	go ji berry	tonifies blood
Lycopus lucidus	ze lan	marsh orchid	vitalizes blood
Lygodium japonicum	jin sha teng	climbing fern	clears heat, cleans toxins
Magnetitum	ci shi	loadstone lode	settles the spirit
Margarite	zhen zhu	pearl	settles the spirit
Margaritifera	zhen zhu mu	mother of pearl	settles the spirit
Malva verticillata	dong kui zi	mallow seed	drains damp
Melia toosendan	chuan lian zi	pagoda tree seed	expel sparasites
Mentha	bo he	mint	releases exterior, cools
Morus alba	sang shen	mulberry	tonifies blood
Morus alba	sang zhi	mulberry branch	dispels wind damp
Morus alba	sang bai pi	mulberry root bark	relieves coughing, wheezing
Morus alba	sang ye	mulberry leaf	releases exterior, cools (leaf)
Oldenlandia diffusae	bai hua she she	Oldenlandia	clears heat, cleans toxins

Ophiopogon japonicus	*men dong*	Ophiopogon	tonifies yin
Oryza sativa	*gu ya*	rice sprout	relieves food stagnation
Ostrera concha	*mu li*	oyster shell	settles the spirit
Paeonia lactiflora	*bai shao*	white peony root	tonifies blood
Paeonia obovata	*chi shao*	red peony root	vitalizes blood
Panax ginseng	*ren shen*	ginseng	tonifies Qi
Panax quinquefolius	*xi yang shen*	American ginseng	tonifies yin
Papaver somniferum	*ying su ke*	opium poppy	astringent
Patrinia scabiosaefolia,	*bai jiang cao*	Patrinia	clears heat, cleans toxins
Perilla frutescens	*zi su ye*	shiso leaf	releases exterior, warms
Perilla frutescens	*su zi*	shiso seed	relieves coughing, wheezing
Persica semen	*tao ren*	peach kernel	vitalizes blood
Pharbitis nil	*qian niu zi*	morning glory seed	draining, harsh expellants
Phaseolus angularis	*chi xiao dou*	adzuki bean	drains damp
Phaseolus radiatus	*lu dou*	mung bean	relieve summer heat
Phellodendron amu-rense	*huang bai*	amur cork tree	clears heat, dries damp
Phragmites communis	*lu gen*	reed	clears heat, drains fire
Phyllostachys nigra	*zhu li*	black bamboo	transforms hot phlegm
Phyllostachys nigra	*zhu ru*	bamboo sap	transforms hot phlegm
Phytolacca acinosa	*shang lu*	asian pokeweed	draining, harsh expellants

Pinellia ternata	*ban xia*	half-summer	transforms cold phlegm
Platyocodon grandiflorum	*jie geng*	balloon flower root	transforms cold phlegm
Polygonatum sibiricum	*huang jing*	yellow essence	tonifies Qi
Polygonatum odoratum	*yu zhu*	Solomon's seal	tonifies yin
Polygonum aviculare	*bian xu*	knotweed	drains damp
Polygonum multiflorum	*he shou wu*	fleeceflower root	tonifies blood
Polygonum multiflorum	*ye jiao teng*	fleeceflower twig	nourishes heart, calms spirit
Polygonum tinctorium	*da qing ye*	Japanese indigo	clears heat, cleans toxins
Poncirus trifoliata	*zhi shi*	trifoliate orange	regulates Qi
Poria cocos	*fu ling*	Hoelen fungus	drains damp
Portulaca oleracea	*ma chi xian*	purslane	clears heat, cleans toxins
Prunella vulgaris	*xia ku cao*	self heal	clears heat, drain fire
Prunus Armeniacae	*xing ren*	almond kernel	relieves coughing, wheezing
Prunus japonica	*yu li ren*	bush cherry pit	draining, moist laxative
Prunus persica	*tao ren*	peach seed	vitalizes blood
Pseudostellaria	*tai zi shen*	'prince' ginseng	tonifies Qi
Pueraria lobata	*ge gen*	kudzu root	releases exterior, cools
Pulsatilla chinensis	*bai tou weng*	anemone root	clears heat, cleans toxins

Raphanus sativus	*lai fu zi*	radish seed	relieves food stagnation
Rehmannia glutinosa	*sheng di*	foxglove root, raw	clears heat, cools blood
Rehmannia glut. prep	*shu di*	foxglove root, cooked	tonifies blood
Rheum	*da huang*	rhubarb rhizome	purgative
Rosa laevigata	*jin ying zi*	cherokee rose	astringent
Rosa rugosa	*mei gui hua*	Chinese tea rose	regulates Qi
Salvia miltiorrhiza	*dan shen*	Chinese sage root	vitalizes blood
Sanguisorba officinalis	*di yu*	burnet	stops bleeding
Saposhnikova divaricata	*fang feng*	siler	releases exterior, warms
Saussurea lappa	*mu xiang*	costus root	regulates Qi
Schizonepeta tenuifolia	*jing jie*	Schizonepeta	releases exterior, warms
Scrophularia ningpoensis	*xuan shen*	ningpo figwort	clears heat, cools blood
Scutellaria baicalensis	*huang qin*	Scutellaria	clears heat, dries damp
Scutellaria barbata	*ban zhi lian*	barbed skullcap	clears heat, cleans toxins
Siegesbeckia orientalis	*xi xian cao*	Siegesbeckia	dispels wind damp
Smilax glabra	*tu fu ling*	glabrous greenbrier	clears heat, cleans toxins
Sophora flavescens	*ku shen*	bitter root	clears heat, dries damp
Stemona japonica	*bai bu*	Stemona root	relieves coughing, wheezing

Squama Manitis	*sang piao xiao*	mantis egg case	astringent
Talcum	*hua shi*	talcum powder	drains damp
Taraxaci mongolici	*pu gong yin*	dandelion	clears heat, cleans toxins
Tetrapanax papyriferus	*tong cao*	rice paper pith	drains damp
Trichosanthes kirilowii	*gua lou*	Trichosanthes fruit	transforms hot phlegm
Trichosanthes kirilowii	*tian hua fen*	heavenly flower	transforms hot phlegm
Tussilago farfara	*kuan dong hua*	coltsfoot	relieves coughing, wheezing
Vaccaria segetalis	*wang bu liu xing*	Vaccaria seed	vitalizes blood
Xanthium sibiricum	*cang er zi*	cocklebur fruit	dispels wind, damp
Zea mays	*yu mi xu*	cornsilk	drains damp
Zingiber officinale	*gan liang*	ginger dried	warms interior, expels cold
Zingiber officinalis	*sheng jiang*	ginger fresh	releases exterior, warms
Zizyphus jujuba	*da zao*	jujube fruit	tonifies Qi
Zizyphus spinosa	*suan zao ren*	jujube fruit seed	nourishes heart, calms spirit

Appendix 2

The Organs: Their Functions, Correspondences, and Characteristics

When you look at the following expressions quickly, they might sound like odd flights of imagination. When you reflect on them, however, you may be able to sense and understand their meaning and their inherent logic. All students of Chinese medicine must memorize these as statements of fact.

The Five Viscera

Heart

Tongue is the portal
Sweat is the fluid
Joy is the emotion
Governs the blood and vessels
Circulates the blood

Governs speech
Irritated by heat
Connected to the small intestine
Home to the *shen* (God, mind, supreme being)
Correspondences: fire, red, bitter flavor

Spleen

Mouth and lips are the portal
Drool is the fluid
Consternation/worry is the emotion
Governs transformation of food into blood and energy
Manages blood
Governs muscles and flesh
Governs the center
Averse to dampness
Connected to the tomach.
Correspondences: earth, yellow, sweet flavor

Lungs

Nose is the portal
Snivel is the fluid
Sorrow or grief is the emotion
Governs Qi of the whole body
Governs the pores, skin, and hair
Governs speech
Sends the Qi downward to the other organs
Governs the defensive exterior
Governs the movement of water in the upper body
Averse to cold
When lungs are well, the nose can tell foul from fragrant
Connected to the large intestine
Correspondences: metal, white, acrid flavor

Kidneys

Ears are the portal
Fluid is urine
Stores the essence of life
Generates Qi
Governs the bones, brain, and marrow
Teeth are the surplus of the bones
Controls the fire of the gate of life
Averse to dryness
Low back is their domain
Connected to the urinary bladder.
Correspondences: water, black, salty taste, winter season

Liver

Eyes are the portal
Tears are the fluid
Emotion is anger
Sensitive to all emotion
Governs discharge
Stores the blood
Governs the joints and tendons
When blood is full in the liver, the sinews can stretch
Governs physical movement
The liver is averse to wind
When the liver is well, the eyes can see the five colors
Correspondences: wood, green-blue, spring season

The Six Bowels

Stomach

Governs intake of food
Governs decomposition
Directs the digestate downward

Enjoys moisture, loathes dryness
Correspondences: see spleen

Small Intestine

Transforms food
Governs absorption
Separates clear and clouded fluids
Correspondences: see heart

Large Intestine

Governs passage, transformation, elimination of waste
Governs liquids
Correspondences: see lungs

Urinary Bladder

Governs the waterworks
Conducts water
Correspondences: see kidneys

Gallbladder

Residence of the clear fluids
Governs decision making
Directs the other organs
Correspondences: see liver

Triple Burner (San Jiao)

Has a name but no form
Governs the sluices
The upper burner governs intake
The middle burner governs transformation
The lower burner governs exiting

Appendix 3

The Processing and Purity of Chinese Herbs

How Herbs Are Processed

Chinese herbal supplements are produced from fresh or dried plants, plant parts, animals, or minerals. Some substances may be collected from the wild, but most are cultivated on farms or in community gardens. Cultivation allows breeding for desirable properties or high yields of selected chemical constituents. However, new varieties may be unpredictable since they lack the track record of strains used for centuries.

Most herbologists consider plants gathered from wildcrafting (gathering plants not specifically planted) to be more natural and more potent than cultivated plants. Herbs gathered in the wild are also free of pesticides and fungicides that may be present in cultivated varieties. Unfortunately, the practice of wild-crafting herbs, along with deforestation, has caused some wild plant species to become endangered.

Many plants are cultivated by pharmaceutical companies. For example, rice yeast is now cultivated to produce statin drugs such as

Lipitor®, yams are grown for steroids, foxglove for digitalis, bella-
donna for atropine, and opium to manufacture morphine. Since processing and harvesting herbs is labor intensive, major cultivators tend
to be places where labor costs are low: China, India, Thailand, South
Korea, Brazil, Mexico, Egypt, Indonesia, Nepal, the Philippines, Kenya,
and Eastern Europe.

Processing Steps

Cleaning of Raw Materials Plants are cleaned after they are harvested. This involves washing, screening, peeling, or stripping leaves.
Unneeded parts are removed before drying.

Drying Plants contain about 60 to 80 percent water when harvested and must contain less than 15 percent when stored. Drying
reduces the water content, enabling the herb to be stored. Plants must
be dried quickly to avoid infestation or spoilage. They can be dried by
both natural and artificial methods.

Natural Drying The oldest method is sun-drying, spreading the herbs
out to dry in the sun or shade. This method requires no equipment, but
uses large amounts of space, and leaves the plants vulnerable to weather.
To save space and protect against inclement weather, drying frames are
sometimes used to air-dry plants in barns or sheds. This method is very
labor intensive and takes much longer than sun or shade drying.

Artificial Drying Artificial dryers reduce drying time and save labor.
Fans blowing unheated air over the herbs can reduce drying time from
weeks to days. Warm-air drying, usually used for medicinal plants, can
take mere hours. There are two types of warm-air dryers: the chamber
dryer, which blows warm air across plants placed in a chamber, and
conveyor dryers, where plants on a conveyor belt pass through a flow
of warm air. Though they are more expensive to house and maintain,
conveyor dryers operate continuously and have very high output.

Cleaning and Sorting When dry, plants are inspected and cleaned
to remove any non-herbal matter. Sand is removed pneumatically.

Metals and stones are removed magnetically and by inspection. Plants are then sorted by size and grade. The highest grades are packaged and sold whole. Lesser grades undergo processing to extract their precious constituents.

Extracting Extraction is the process of removing the chemical constituents of a plant by using a solvent. Plants are ground up and mixed with a chemical solvent such as alcohol, vinegar, glycerin, hexane, or benzene, depending on which constituents are being extracted, the cost, and environmental issues. The resulting liquid containing the dissolved substance is called the miscella.

Liquid Extract (Miscella) Using Solvents The techniques for solvent extraction are maceration, percolation, and counter-current extraction. Maceration involves soaking and agitating the solvent and plant materials together. The solvent is then drained and the remaining miscella is removed through pressing or centrifuging. With percolation, the plant matter is placed in a series of chambers where it repeatedly percolates with a solvent until the active ingredients have been leached into the solvent. Counter-current extraction, possibly the most effective method, involves the solvent flowing in a current against the plant material. This method is continuous, unlike the other methods, which are batch processes.

Miscella can contain unwanted substances such as tannins, pigments, microbial contaminants, or solvent residue. These impurities are removed by decanting, filtration, sedimentation, centrifuging, heating, adsorption, precipitation, or ion exchange. Sometimes the raw, unprocessed miscella is used as the medicine. This is called a "fluid extract."

The miscella can be further concentrated through evaporation or vaporization with mild heat. The miscella should not be heated too much because it can be degraded by heat.

Powdered Extract Powdered extracts are less subject to microbial contamination than are liquid extracts. Such powdered extracts do not require refrigeration and can more easily be stored for longer periods of time. Powders usually require the addition of excipient substances (inactive substances used as a carrier for the active ingredients of the medicine). Common excipients are corn or rice starch, cellulose, maltodextrin, or other simple sugars. Vacuum freeze dryers, cabinet vacuum dryers, continuously operating drum or belt dryers, microwave ovens, and atomizers are all used to dry extracts and make powders from the liquid miscella.

Extraction with Gases This method exposes plant matter to a gas under high pressure, dissolving the active ingredients. Gases such as carbon dioxide, nitrogen, methane, ethane, ethylene, nitrous oxide, sulfur dioxide, propane, propylene, ammonia, and sulfur hexafluoride are all used for differing circumstances. This method uses lower temperatures, preserving components normally degraded by heat.

Steam Distillation Steam is injected from underneath the plant material, dissolving substances in the plant. The steam, saturated with the dissolved matter, then enters a condenser where it is cooled back into a liquid. The extract either rises to the top or settles to the bottom of the liquid and is then separated from the water.

Cold Pressing This process extracts essential oils through pressing. Known as enfleurage, it is used to make perfume from flowers. This method uses purified fats to extract essential plant components. Plant material is simply spread onto sheets of purified fat, which then dissolve the essential ingredients.

Decoctions and Infusions Decoctions are water extracts where herbs are boiled for three minutes to one hour. Ceramic or tempered glass pots are preferred for boiling, but stainless steel can also be used. Never use aluminum, iron, or copper vessels to boil herbs, as these elements will enter the decoction, altering the properties of the medicine. Decocted liquids require refrigeration. Infusions are made by soaking herbs in hot water, as when preparing tea, to dissolve the active ingredients. As with decoctions, the infused liquid must be refrigerated.

For medicinal oils, herbs are simply soaked in an oil, such as sesame, almond, peanut, or olive.

Potential Impurities in Herbs

Many have expressed concern about impurities in Chinese medicines. In April 2003, there was a scare when the California Department of Health Services tested a variety of imported Chinese patent medicines and found many impurities, unlisted ingredients, endangered species, and false statements.

Well aware of these problems, Dr. Shen's was manufacturing these patent medicines itself, specifically so that it could oversee the manufacturing, scrutinize and test every herb, and be 100 percent confident of the correctness and quality of the ingredients.

It should be noted that the government of China, having recognized the emerging world markets for Chinese medicine, has undertaken far-reaching efforts to modernize this industry. In July 2001, China adopted the "Green Trade Standards of Importing and Exporting Medicinal Plants and Preparations," which mandates testing for pesticides, heavy metals, bacteria, and the like.

Importers of herbal medicines have also become far more discriminating about which medicines to import. Thus, the imported patent medicines available to consumers today are far more pure and safe today than they were ten years ago. Nevertheless, for those who are concerned, following is a comprehensive list of possible impurities in herbal medicines.

Heavy Metals

On many bottles of herbal medicines you will find the following warning: *This product contains lead, an element known by the state of California to cause cancer, birth defects, and other reproductive harm.*

Rest assured, these products are safe, and don't caused cancer, birth defects, or reproductive harm. The problem is Proposition 65, The California Safe Drinking Water and Toxic Enforcement Act of 1986. Among other things, it restricted the amounts of heavy metals allowable in food and water to levels far lower than any previously established. Though these elements occur naturally in food and water, excessive exposure can cause birth defects and some kinds of cancers. Few Chinese herbal medicines today contain much heavy metal. Arsenic and mercury have been removed as medicinal ingredients.

The only issue with herbal products is trace amounts of lead. Governments and other organizations have declared varying amounts of lead to be acceptable in medicinal herbal products. Japan allows twenty parts per million for total metals in herbal medicines, and the World Health Organization allows ten. Both Germany and the Australian Therapeutic Goods Administration allow five parts per million of lead in a product. The U.S. Pharmacopoeia has no standards for herbs, but allows three parts per million in drugs.

Most Chinese herbal products test at an average of one to three parts per million. However, California's Proposition 65 requires a warning for just one-half part per million in food, and medicinal herbs are considered food in California. This extremely low level set for food or water is inappropriate for herbal medicines, which should be rich with naturally occurring minerals. Proposition 65 allows the sale of these products, but requires a warning.

Pesticides

Many Chinese herbs are collected in the wild and contain no trace of pesticides. Some plants have been bred to be resistant to pests and do not require the use of pesticides. However, some cultivated herbs are grown with pesticides or fungicides. All Chinese herb growers are sensitive to this issue and take precautions to avoid contamination in harvested plants. Traces of pesticides have occasionally been found in these cultivated varieties.

However, pesticide use may be far less common than is thought. Many cultivators don't use chemical pesticides because in China, fertilizers and pesticides are expensive while labor is cheap. Many cultivators rely instead on hand removal of pests, cheaper natural agents, and more meticulous cultivation.

The Chinese are not enamored of poisons, and regulations in China require cultivators to use techniques that minimize pesticide residues.

Ginseng cultivation is the best example. Fungicides are used, at times, because ginseng is susceptible to infestation. However, farmers avoid applying these chemicals near harvest time so that wind and rain have time to blow and wash away the fungicides before the harvest.

Fumigants (pesticides applied after harvest) Some people believe that Chinese herbs are routinely fumigated at American ports. This is absolutely not true. Many tons of herbs have been imported each year for many years. None have ever been fumigated on either side of the Pacific. The U.S. Department of Agriculture and Food and Drug Administration also deny that this is commonly done. Sometimes, when herbs are warehoused for an abnormally long period of time due to a delay in distribution, some fumigants might be used. However, consumers should not be concerned, as many of these fumigants are actually herbal rather than chemical. Also, the distribution of Chinese herbs is efficient; herbs are rarely delayed, so they almost never need fumigants.

Chinese herbs imported into the United States rarely show signs of infestation and are usually far cleaner than herbs imported from other parts of the world. Western herbs frequently come from Mexico, South or Central America, and Eastern Europe. They also might be fumigated during storage.

Sulfur

Sulfur is prevalent throughout the human body and is essential for life. Several Chinese herbs have relatively high levels of sulfur. This is deliberate. The sulfur comes from a processing method where herbs are smoked with heated sulfur. The resulting residues, though they are sulfites, do not appear to cause reactions in sulfite-sensitive people. Sulfur is used on herbs that are moist or those that discolor significantly. Sulfur is also a Chinese herb used for topical infections, and is taken internally in small amounts to build kidney yang.

Irradiation

Most of the spices sold in grocery stores are sterilized by ionizing radiation. Except for certain animal materials, Chinese herbs are not irradiated. Deer antlers and other animal parts are irradiated under direction of the U.S. Department of Agriculture to assure that disease-causing viral and other organisms are not present. Irradiation does not make herbs radioactive or leave traces of radiation. Some manufacturers may use gamma irradiation to reduce bacteria counts in their products; this also causes no radioactive contamination.

Sterilizing Gas Residue

Another way to reduce bacteria count is to sterilize herbs with a gas, such as ethylene oxide, which may result in ethylene residue. As virtually all treated bacteria are harmless, there is no evidence that sterilizing the herbs is necessary in almost any case. This technique might be employed in the very rare instance that harmful bacteria are found.

Bacteria, Mold, Yeast, and Other Organisms

For the most part, herbs are free of harmful bacteria. Salmonella, the bacteria that can cause most food poisoning, is not found in Chinese herb formulas. Likewise, toxic strains of E-coli, an indicator of fecal contamination, is almost never found in Chinese herbs. Counts of harmless bacteria in Chinese herb tablets are usually considered low.

Western Drugs in Chinese Patent Medicines

Some imported Chinese patent medicines contain ingredients not listed on the label. These unlisted ingredients can include Western drugs. One case in point is the sugar-coated variety of *yin chiao* from Tianjin, which includes an analgesic and an antihistamine (it also has added caffeine). None of these ingredients appear on the label. Other common drug additives include aspirin, acetaminophen, antihistamines, and antibiotics.

Additives

Chinese pills may be coated with sugar or vegetable oil, or made with honey. Most cough syrups and liquid extracts are made with sugar and honey. Flow agents, binders, and coatings are used just as they are in the West. Tablets and capsules may also have artificial colors added.

Granulated herbs usually contain a starch or sugar base, such as potato or corn starch or malt dextrin. This allows the granulated herb to be dissolved in liquid. In most cases, these additions comprise less than 15 percent of the granulated powder. Certain oily herbs, however, require a much higher percentage of these additives. In a few cases, added sugars constitute as much as 50 percent of the product.

Wrong Herb Used

Substitution of herbs is routinely practiced in Chinese medicine. This is usually done because of herb availability or cost. Rarely does such a substitution cause harm, but using the wrong herb is another matter. In the most publicized incident to date about Chinese herbs, an herb was thought to be the cause of liver damage.

Actually the culprit was incompetence, not on the part of an herbologist, but of a group of Belgian MDs in a 1993 weight loss study. They used the wrong herb, replacing a harmless herb with a toxic cousin. The offending herb contained aristolochic acid and was suspected of causing liver damage. Oddly, the doctors were not held responsible by the press or public, and their competence was never questioned. Instead, the herb was blamed.

Some substitutions are actually labeling errors, intentional or otherwise. Occasionally, herbs are named in a product but are not actually contained in the product. Products using the word "ginseng" in their name frequently use *dang shen* ("poor man's ginseng") instead. Tiger bone, musk, rhinoceros horn, and other endangered species do not actually exist in products bearing their names; chemicals or other herbs with similar properties are substituted. None of the medicines listing these endangered species and tested by the U.S. Fish and Wildlife Department actually contained them.

Appendix 4

Food as Medicine

Modern medicine seems to ignore the obvious: foods can stimulate body processes and potentially trigger (or relieve) countless pathologic events such as inflammation, fever, hyperactivity, or hormonal abnormalities. Organs and Qi are negatively affected by dietary extremes such as those commonly seen in modern developed nations, such as overeating and eating too many stimulating foods. Correcting such extremes can have a positive effect on health.

The effects of overeating, obesity, diabetes, and the like are well known, but the effects of an overly-stimulating diet are not understood at all. Such patterns might appear as fevers, sweats, insomnia, hyperthyroid, or inflammatory skin conditions. Over-consumption of foods considered hot, stimulating, or yang in nature will worsen these sumptoms. Over-stimulated people may benefit from foods that are considered cool, calming, or yin.

Conversely, those who have cold or yang deficient conditions, such as fatigue, feeling cold, low blood pressure, hypersomnia, sciatica, hypothyroid, or Hashimoto's complex, may do better with a more stimulating (yang) diet.

Cooking can effect how stimulating foods are. Hotter cooking methods like barbecuing or frying will create a more stimulating (yang) food. Cooler cooking methods like boiling or steaming will result in cooler (yin) foods.

The following list reflects Chinese diets, so some common Western foods may be absent. The occasional disagreement among sources on whether a food is cool, neutral, or hot is marked below with asterisks. When altering your diet, make moderation the rule. Changes are most sustainable when they are introduced gradually.

Stimulating (Yang)	Neutral	Calming (Yin)
Apricots*	Almonds	Yogurt
Artichoke	Apples**	Abalone
Basil	Artichoke	Agar
Beef*	Jerusalem	Banana
Black Tea	Artichoke	Barley
Butter	Beans, kidney**	Beer
Butterfish	Bean Sprouts	Beans**
Carp*	Beets	Bean curd**
Cayenne	Black Mushrooms	Bran
Celery*	Blueberries	Buckwheat
Cherries	Cabbage	Cottage Cheese
Chestnuts	Carrots	Crab
Chicken	Catfish	Cucumber
Chili	Cauliflower	Duck**
Cinnamon	Carob	Eggplant
Chives	Cheese	Egg, white
Coconut	Clams**	Frog's legs
Coconut Milk	Coconut oil	Gluten
Cod	Corn	Kelp
Coffee	Currant	Lettuce
Coriander	Eel	Lotus root
Dates	Figs	Malt
Egg, yolk	Guava	Mango
	Grits	

Fennel	Honey	Marrow
Garlic	Huckleberries	Melon
Ginger	Mackerel	Millet
Goose*	Maple Syrup	Mulberries
Grapes*	Milk	Mung Beans
Green Onion	Nutmeg	Mushrooms
Ham	Okra	Octopus
Lamb	Olive Oil	Oysters
Malt	Papaya	Pears
Mussels	Peanuts	Peas
Mustard	Pecans	
Mustard Greens	Perch	
Nectarine	Pinto Beans	
Oats	Pork	
Olives	Potatoes	
Onions	Pumpkin Seeds	
Oolong Tea	Quail	
Parsley	Raisin*	
Peach	Rice	
Pepper	Sardines	
Pineapple*	Sesame Seeds	
Pine Nut	Shark	
Plums*	Shitake Mushroom	
Safflower	Sugar, white	
Shrimp	Strawberries	
Soy oil	String Bean	
Sugar, brown	Sturgeon	
Sweet Potato	Tapioca	
Turkey	Taro	
Turmeric	Turnip	
Vinegar	Vanilla	
Walnuts	Whitefish	
Wine	Winter Squash	
	Yam	
	Yogurt	

* Classified in some texts as stimulating and in others as neutral

**Classified in some texts as calming and in others as neutral

Appendix 5

Resources

Reading List

Beinfield, Harriet, and Efrem Korngold. *Between Heaven and Earth* (New York: Ballantine, 1991).

Bensky, Dan, and Andrew Gamble. *Chinese Herbal Medicine Materia Medica* (Seattle: Eastland Press, 1986).

Bensky, Dan, and Randal Barolet. *Chinese Herbal Medicine Formulas and Strategies* (Seattle: Eastland Press, 1990).

Butt, Gary, and Frena Bloomfield. *Harmony Rules: The Chinese Way of Health Through Food* (York Beach, Maine: Samuel Weiser, 1987).

Cohen, Misha Ruth, and Kaliea Doner. *The Chinese Way to Healing: Many Paths to Wholeness* (New York: Perigree, 1996).

Duo Gao. *Chinese Medicine* (New York: Thunder's Mouth Press, 1997).

Eisenberg, David. *Encounters With Qi* (New York: W.W. Norton, 1985).

Ellis, Andrew, Nigel Wiseman, and Ken Boss. *Fundamentals of Chinese Acupuncture* (Brookline, Mass: Paradigm Publications, 1988).

Flaws, Bob, Charles Chace, and Michael Helme. *Timing and the Times, Chronicity in the American Practice of Oriental Medicine* (Boulder, Colorado: Blue Poppy Press, 1986).

Fratkin, Jake. *Chinese Herbal Patent Formulas* (Portland, Oregon: Institute For Traditional Medicine, 1986).

Fung, Dr. Fung, and John Fung. *Sixty Years in Search of Cures* (Dublin, California: Get Well Foundation, 1994).

Gaeddert, Andrew. *Chinese Herbs in the Western Clinic* (Dublin, California: Get Well Foundation, 1994).

Kaptchuk, Ted. *The Web That Has No Weaver* (New York: Congdon & Reed, 1983).

Leslie, Charles. *Asian Medical Systems* (Berkeley, California: University of California Press, 1976).

Lu, Henry. *Chinese System of Food Cures* (New York: Sterling, 1986).

McNamara, Sheila. *Traditional Chinese Medicine* (New York, New York: Basic Books, 1995).

Porkert, Manfred. *Essentials of Chinese Diagnosis* (Zurich, Switzerland: Chinese Medicine Publications, 1983).

Reid, Daniel. *The Complete Book of Chinese Health and Healing* (Boston: Shambala, 1994).

Reid, Daniel. *Chinese Herbal Medicine* (Boston: Shambala, 1996).

Rogans, Eve. *Chinese Herbal Medicine: A Step-By-Step Guide* (Rockport, Masachussetts: Element, 1994).

Teegarden, Ron. *Chinese Tonic Herbs* (New York: Japan Publications, 1984).

Tierra, Lesley. *Healing with Chinese Herbs* (Freedom, California: Crossing Press, 1997).

Unschuld, Paul. *Medicine in China: History of Ideas* (Berkeley, California: University of California Press, 1985).

Wallnofer, Heinrich, and Anna Von Rottauscher. *Chinese Folk Medicine and Acupuncture*, translated by Marion Palmedo (New York, New York: Bell Publishing, 1965).

Wicke, Roger. *Traditional Chinese Herbal Science Volume 1, The Language and Patterns of Life, 5th edition*, Online Version, Chapters 1–6 (Hot Springs, Montana: Rocky Mountain Herbal Institute, 1994).

Wicke, Roger. *Traditional Chinese Herbal Science Volume 2, Herbs, Strategies and Case Studies, 4th edition* (Hot Springs, Montana: Rocky Mountain Herbal Institute, 1994).

Wiseman, Nigel. *Glossary of Chinese Medicine* (Brookline, Massachusetts: Paradigm Publications, 1990).

Yeung, Him-Che. *Handbook of Chinese Herbs and Formulas* (Los Angeles: Institute of Chinese Medicine, 1985).

Zhu, Chun-Lan. *Clinical Handbook of Prepared Chinese Medicines* (Brookline Massachusetts: Paradigm Press, 1989).

U.S. Schools of Chinese Medicine

Academy of Chinese Culture and Health Sciences
1601 Clay Street
Oakland, CA 94612
Tel: (510) 763-7787
Fax: (510) 834-8646

Academy of Oriental Medicine
P.O. Box 9446,
Austin, TX 78766-9446
Tel: (512) 454-1188
Fax: (512) 454-7001
E-mail: ACUAOMA@aol.com

Acupuncture and Herbal Medicine College
Tai Hsuan Foundation
2600 S. King Street, #206
Honolulu, HI 96726
P.O. Box 11130
Honolulu, HI 96728-0130
Tel: (800) 942-4788
Voice: (808) 949-1050
Fax: (808) 949-1005
E-mail: taihsuan@acupuncture-hi.com

Acupuncture and Integrative Medicine College, Berkeley
2550 Shattuck Avenue,
Berkeley, CA 94704
Tel: (510) 666-8248 x106
E-mail: admissions@aimc.edu
Website: www.aimc.edu

American Academy of Acupuncture and Oriental Medicine
1925 West County Road B2
Roseville, MN 55113
Tel: (651) 631-0204
Website: www.aaaom.org

American College of Acupuncture
9100 Park West Drive
Houston, TX 77063
Tel: (800) 729-4456, (713) 780-9777
FAX: (713) 781-5781
E-mail: acaom@compuserve.com
Website: www.acaom.edu

American College of Traditional Chinese Medicine
455 Arkansas Street
San Francisco, CA 94107
Tel: (415) 282-7600
Fax: (415) 282-0856

Atlantic Institute of Oriental Medicine
1057 SE 17th St.
Ft. Lauderdale, FL 33316
Tel: (954) 463-3888, (954) 522-6405

Bastyr University
14500 Juanita Drive NE
Bothell, WA 98011
Tel: (206) 823-1300
Fax: (206) 823-6222
Acupuncture and Oriental Medicine Department: (206) 602-3120

Chinese Medicine and Acupuncture Institute
8102 West Chester Pike
Upper Darby, PA 19082
Tel: (610) 789-7898
E-mail: Martyeisen@aol.com

Chinese Healing Arts Center
73-3 Great Plains Rd.
Danbury, CT 06811
Phone: (914) 687-0988
Fax: (203) 791-9980
E-mail: QiHealer@aol.com

Colorado School of Acupuncture and
Oriental Medicine, Inc.
2755 S. Locust St. # 200
Denver, CO 80222
Tel: (303) 757-4438
E-mail: csaom@earthlink.net

Colorado School of Traditional Chinese Medicine
1441 York Street, Suite 202
Denver, CO 80206
Tel: (303) 329-6355

Community School of Traditional Chinese Healthcare
1190 N.E. 125 th Street, #12
North Miami, FL 33161

Emperor's College of Traditional Oriental Medicine
1807-B Wilshire Blvd.
Santa Monica, CA 90403
Tel: (310) 453-8300
Fax: (310) 829-3838

Five Branches Institute: College of
Traditional Chinese Medicine
200 7th Ave.
Santa Cruz, CA 95062
Tel: (408) 476-9424
Fax: (408) 476-8928

Florida Health Academy
261 Ninth St. South
Naples, FL 34102
Tel: (941) 495-8282, (941) 263-9391

Florida Institute of Traditional Chinese Medicine
5335 66th St. North
St. Petersburg, FL 33709
Tel: (813) 546-6565, (800) 565-1246

Florida School of Acupuncture and Oriental Medicine
1705 NW 6th Street
Gainesville, FL 32609
Tel: (352) 371-2833
Fax: (352) 371-2867
E-mail: Dbole@aol.com

Green Mountain Institute of Acupuncture
and Holistic Medicine
P. O. Box 4547
White River Junction, VT 05001
Tel: (802) 295-2603

Institute of Chinese Herbology
At-Home Study Program
8 Charles Hill Circle
Orinda, CA 94563
Tel: (800) 736-0182
Website: ich-herbschool.com

Institute of Chinese Medicine
2507 Ennalls Avenue, Suite 203
Wheaton, MD 20902
Tel: (301) 929-68-55
Fax: (301) 445-3258
(301) 406-4933

Institute of Clinical Acupuncture and Oriental Medicine
1270 Queen Emma Street #107
Honolulu, HI 96813
Tel/Fax : (808) 521-2288
E-mail: ICAOM@msn.com

International Institute of Chinese Medicine
P.O. Box 4991
Santa Fe, NM 87502
Tel: (505) 473-5233
Fax: (505) 473-9279

Albuquerque Branch Campus:
4600 Montgomery, NE, Bldg. 1, Ste. 1,
Albuquerque, NM 87109
Tel: (505) 883-5569
Fax: (505) 883-5569

International College of Traditional Chinese Medicine of Vancouver
Suite 201, 1508 W. Broadway,
Vancouver, B.C. Canada V6J 1W8
Tel: (604) 731-2926
Fax: (604) 731-2964
E-mail: info@tcmcollege.com

Jung Tao School of Classical Chinese Medicine
207 Dale Adams Road
Sugar Grove NC 28679
Tel: (828) 297-4181
E-mail: info@jungtao.com
Website: www.jungtao.edu

Keimyung Baylo University
1126 N. Brookhurst Street
Anaheim, CA 92801
Tel: (714) 533-1495
Fax: (714) 533-6040
E-mail: webinfo@kbu.edu

Los Angeles Branch Campus:
2727 W 6th St.
Los Angeles, CA 90015
Tel: (213) 738-0712
Fax: (213) 480-1332

Kyung San University
8322 Garden Grove Blvd.
Garden Grove, CA 92644
Tel: (714) 636-3445
fax: (714) 636-0337
E-mail: admin@kyungsan.edu

London College of Traditional Acupuncture & Oriental Medicine
Tel: +44 208 371 0820
E-mail: college@lcta.com
Website: www.lcta.com

Maryland Institute of Traditional Chinese Medicine
4641 Montgomery Ave. Suite 415
Bethesda, MD 20814
Tel: (301) 718-7373
Fax: (301) 718-0735

Mercy College
555 Broadway
Dobbs Ferry, NY 10522
Admissions: 1-800-MERCY NY
Tel: (800) 637-2969
Program office: (914) 674-7401
E-mail: admissions@merlin.mercynet.edu

Midwest Center for the Study of Oriental Medicine
6226 Bankers Road Suites 5 & 6
Racine, WI 53403
Tel: (414) 554-2010
Fax: (414) 554-7475
Chicago Branch Campus:
4334 N. Hazel #206
Chicago, IL 60613
Tel: (773) 975-1295
E-mail: 75703.3001@compuserve.com

Minnesota College of Acupuncture and Oriental Medicine
at Northwestern Health Sciences University.
2501 W. 84th St. Bloomington, MN 55431
Tel: (952) 888-4777

National Institute of Oriental Medicine
7100 Lake Ellenor Drive
Orlando, FL 32809
Tel: (407) 888-8689
Fax: (407) 888-8211
E-Mail: niom@tesi.net

The New Center College for Wholistic
Health Education and Research
6801 Jericho Turnpike
Syosset, NY 11791-4465
Tel: (516) 364-0808
Fax: (516) 364-0989

Oregon College of Oriental Medicine
10525 SE Cherry Blossom Dr.
Portland, OR 97216
Tel: (503) 253-3443
Fax: (503) 253-2701

Pacific College of Oriental Medicine
7445 Mission Valley Rd. Suites 103-106
San Diego, CA 92108
Tel: (619) 574-6909
Fax: (619) 574-6641
E-mail: admissions-sd@pacificcollege.edu

Chicago Branch Campus:
3646 N. Broadway, 2nd Floor
Chicago, IL 60613
Tel: (888) 729-4811
Fax: (773) 477-4109

Pacific Institute of Oriental Medicine, New York
915 Broadway, 3rd Floor
New York, NY 10010
Tel: (212) 982-3456
Fax: (212) 982-6641
E-mail: jmiller@ormed.edu
Website: www.pacificcollege.edu

Phoenix Institute of Herbal Medicine & Acupuncture (PIHMA)
P.O. Box 2659
Scottsdale, AZ 85252
Tel: (602) 274-1885
Fax: (602) 423-5292
Website: cniemiec@pihma.com

Rain Star University
4110–4130 N. Goldwater Blvd.
Scottsdale, AZ 85251
Tel: (480) 423-0375, Outside AZ (888) RAINSTAR
Fax: (480) 945-9824
E-mail: info@RainStarUniversity.com

Rocky Mountain Herbal Institute
P.O. Box 579
Hot Springs, MT 59845
Tel.: (406) 741-3811
Website: www.rmhiherbal.org

Royal University of America
1125 West 6th St.
Los Angeles, CA 90017
Tel: (213) 482-6646
Fax: (213) 482-6649

Ruseto College
2900 Valmont Rd., E1
Boulder, CO 80301
Tel: (303) 449-1686

Samra University of Oriental Medicine
600 St. Paul Ave.
Los Angeles, CA 90017
Tel: (213) 482-8448
Fax: (213) 482-9020
E-mail: 103346.1422@compuserve.com

Santa Barbara College of Oriental Medicine
1919 State Street, Suite 204
Santa Barbara, CA 93101
Tel: (805) 898-1180
Fax: (805) 682-1864
Email: admissions@SBCOM.edu

The Sarasota School of Natural Healing Arts
8216 South Tamiami Trail
Sarasota, FL 34238
Tel: (941) 966-7117 or (800) 966-7117
E-mail: ssnha@aol.com

Seattle Institute of Oriental Medicine
916 NE 65th, Suite B
Seattle, WA 98115
Tel: (206) 517-4541
Fax: (206) 526-1932

Southwest Acupuncture College
Santa Fe Campus
1622 Galisteo Street
Santa Fe, NM 87505
Tel: (505) 438-8884
Fax: (505) 438-8883
E-mail: SFe@acupuncturecollege.edu

Albuquerque Campus
7801 Academy, NE
Albuquerque, NM 87109
Tel: (505) 888-8898
Fax: (505) 888-1380
E-mail: ABQ@acupuncturecollege.edu

Boulder Branch Campus
6620 Gunpark Drive
Boulder, CO 80301
Tel: (303) 581-9955
Fax: (303) 581-9944
E-mail: Boulder@acupuncturecollege.
Website: www.acupuncturecollege.edu

Southwest College of Naturopathic Medicine
& Health Sciences School of Acupuncture
2140 E. Broadway Road
Tempe, AZ 85282
Tel: (602) 858-9100
Fax: (602) 858-9116

Texas Institute of Traditional Chinese Medicine
4005 Manchaca Road, Suite 200
Austin, TX 78704
Tel: (512) 444-8082
Fax: (512) 346-0987

Third Coast Insitute of Acupuncture and Oriental Medicine
2947 Walnut Hill Lane, #101
Dallas, TX 75229
Tel: (214) 351-6464

Traditional Acupuncture Institute
American City Building
10227 Wincopin Circle, Suite 100
Columbia, MD 21044-3422
Tel: (301) 596-6006
Fax: (410) 964-3544

Traditional Chinese Medical College of Hawaii
Parker Ranch Office Center, Bldg. 3
P.O. Box 2288
Kamuela, HI 96743
Phone/Fax: (808) 885-9226

Tri-State Institute of Traditional Chinese Acupuncture
80 8th Ave., 4th Floor,
New York, NY 10011
Tel: (212) 496-7869
Fax: (212) 496-0648

Worsley Institute of Classical Acupuncture
6175 NW 153rd Street, Suite 324
Miami Lakes, FL 33014
Tel: (305) 823-7270
Fax: (305) 823-6603

YoSan University of Traditional Chinese Medicine
1314 Second Street, Suite 200
Santa Monica, CA 90401
Tel: (310) 917-2202
Fax: (310) 917-2267

Manufacturers of Chinese Medicine

U.S. Manufacturers

Dr. Shen's, 2322 5th St., Berkeley, CA 94710

East Earth Trade Winds, P.O. Box 493151, Redding, CA 96049

Evergreen Herbs, 17431 East Gale Ave, City of Industry, CA 91748

Golden Flower Chinese Herbs, 2724 Vassar Place NE, Albuquerque, NM 87107

Health Concerns, 8001 Capwell Dr., Oakland, CA 94621

Institute for Traditional Medicine, 2017 SE Hawthorne Blvd., Portland, OR 97214

K'an Herb Company, 6001 Butler Ln., Scotts Valley, CA 95066

Planetary Herbal Products, P.O. Box 779, Brookdale, CA 95007

Shen Clinic, 1385 Shattuck Ave., Berkeley, CA 94709

Spring Wind Herbs, Inc., 2325 Fourth Street, Suite 6, Berkeley, CA 94710

Chinese Manufacturers

Anyang Huaan Pharmaceutical, Henan

Bai Yun Pharmaceutical Factory, Guangzhou

Bejing Pharmaceuticals, Beijing

Bio Essence Brand, imported by Bio Essence Corp, Richmond, California

China National Native Produce and Animal-by-Products, Hebei, China

Chung Lien Drug Works, Wuhan

First Factory of Chinese Traditional Medicine, Guangzhou

Fo Shan Herbal Product Company, Guangdong

Fushan United Manufactory, Guangzhou

Guandong Medicine & Health Products, Guangdong

Guilin Chinese Medicine Factory, Guangxi

Handan Pharmaceutical Works, Hebei

Harbin Second Chinese Medicine Factory, Harbin
Herbal Times Brand, imported by Nuherbs, Oakland, California
Huale Herbs Factory, Guangzhou
Huqingyutang Pharmaceutical Factory, Hangzhou
Kwangchhow Pharmaceutical Industry, Guangzhou
Lanzhou Taibo Pharmaceutical Factory, Gansu
Meizhou City Pharmaceuticals, Guangdong
Min-Kang Drug Manufactory, Yinchang
Minshan Brand, by Lanzhou Foci Herb Factory, Lanzhou
National Chemicals Corp., Guangzhou
No. 3 Traditional Chinese Pharmacy Factory, Shanghai
Pangaoshou Pharmaceutical Company, Guangzhou
Peking Medicine Manufactory, Beijing
Peking Tung Jen Tang Manufactory, Beijing
People's Pharmaceutical Factory, Jilin
Plum Flower Brand, imported by May Way, Oakland, California
San Ming Factory, Fujan, China
Shanghai Chinese Medicine Works, Shanghai
Siping Pharmaceutical Works, Jilin
Swatow United Medicine Factory, Shantou
Szechuan Provincial Pharmaceutical Factory, Chengdu
Tai Zhou Pharmaceutical Factory, Zhejiang
Tanglong Gansu Medicines, Lanzhou
Tianjin Brand, manufactured by Tianjin Health Products, Tianjin
Tientsin Drug Manufactory, Tianjin
United Pharmaceutical Manufactory, Guangzhou
Wellconie International Pharmaceutical, Shanghai
Wuhan Zhong Ian Drug Factory, Wuhan
Yu Lam Medicine Factory, Guangdong
Yulin Pharmaceuticals Co., Yulin
Zhonghua Pharmaceuticals Factory, Guangzhou
Zhong Sheng Chinese Medicine Factory, Guangzhou

Glossary

Accumulations are swellings, cysts, or tumors caused by stagnation, poor flow, or excess dampness.

Acupressure is a massage technique using the channels and acupuncture points (see Chapter 1, "Methods of Chinese Medicine").

Acupuncture is the Chinese medical practice of inserting hair-thin needles in the body to heal and relieve pain (see Chapter 1, "Methods of Chinese Medicine").

Acupuncture Points are located all over the body, but primarily on fourteen major pathways or channels. The points are stimulated by needles, heat, or massage to affect the flow of Qi and blood, and thus influence the organs.

Blood is the red liquid that moistens, nourishes, and cleans the cells and organs.

Blood Deficiency is a blood weakness with symptoms of anemia, dizziness, dry skin or hair, scant or absent menstruation, fatigue, pale skin or tongue, and poor memory.

Calms the Spirit, see Settles the Spirit.

Channels, see Meridians.

Cold means decreased activity or function due to lack of heat or yang. Signs of cold include pain, chills, or feeling cold, poor circulation, loose stools or diarrhea, slow pulse, aversion to cold, or a preference for warm beverages.

Damp, dampness consists of excessive fluids with symptoms of abdominal bloating, loss of appetite, nausea, vomiting, lack of thirst, or feeling heavy and fatigued.

Damp Heat is a condition combining dampness and heat. These are often purulent infections, jaundice, or hepatitis.

Decoction is a medicinal beverage made with herbs boiled in water.

Deficiency is any weakness or insufficiency.

Deficiency Heat, see Empty Heat.

Diaphoretic causes sweating.

Diuretic causes urination.

Dry, dryness is a condition caused by lack of yin, blood, or fluids in the body, and is characterized by dry skin, hair, eyes, lips, joints, stool, or lubricating fluids.

Eight Principles are four sets of factors used to apply the theory of yin and yang to the body and to health (see Chapter 3, "Understanding Theories of Chinese Medicine").

Empty Heat is a deficiency of yin or fluids resulting in symptoms such as hot flashes, mood swings, night sweats, and other hormonal changes, and is also known as Deficiency Heat or Empty Fire.

Essence is also known as *jing*. It is a substance affecting the course of reproduction, maturation, and growth. It is considered the foundation of Qi, and it is stored in the kidney.

Excess refers to too much heat, cold, damp, dry, yin, or yang.

Excess Yang is an overactive metabolism with symptoms of heat, rapid pulse, hypertension, aggression, loud voice, or restlessness.

Excess Yin means excessive fluids, often with symptoms of swelling or dampness. Sometimes this condition is caused by the body having heat insufficient to evaporate the fluids.

External is the source of a pathogen or illness coming from outside the body.

External Evils are also known as atmospheric or climatic factors, or evil Qi excess. These include wind, cold, summer heat, dampness, dryness, and fire.

Fire is excess heat energy that is stronger than excess yang. Some symptoms of fire include fever, red eyes, sore throat, flushed face, bleeding, or inflammation.

Five Phases are also known as the five elements or the *wu xing*. This is a theory of nature often used in diagnosing and assessing the patient (see Chapter 3, "Understanding Theories of Chinese Medicine").

Internal means inside the body.

Internal Wind is a condition inside the body that produces spasms or seizures. Includes everything from facial tics to strokes.

Jing, see essence.

Meridians are also called channels. They are the pathways through which Qi flows. The flow of Qi nourishes the body and fows the organs to function.

Organ is a collection of body functions and structures given the name of an internal organ. An organ, according to Chinese medicine, resembles a system in Western medicine. The lung organ, for example, includes many of the functions and body parts that we would assign to the respiratory system (see The Twelve Organs in Chapter 3, "Understanding Theories of Chinese Medicine").

Phlegm is a sticky fluid used by the body for lubrication and excretion.

Qi is energy, the force of nature that creates movement or heat.

Qi Deficiency means low energy, usually resulting in weakness, possibly including symptoms of shortness of breath, slow metabolism, loose stool, frequent colds, weak voice, heart palpitations, or frequent urination.

Qi Gong is a discipline of concentration and movement, used to cultivate and move Qi, to heal and maintain health (see Chapter 1, "Methods of Chinese Medicine").

San Jiao, see Triple Warmer.

Settles the Spirit means it has a sedative or calming effect on the mind and nervous system.

Shen is the spirit, mind, God, or supreme being residing in the heart.

Stagnation is a blockage or excess buildup of Qi or blood that prevents free flow. Stagnation is frequently accompanied by pain, bloating, or accumulations.

Stomach Heat or Fire is an inflamed condition in the stomach with symptoms of bad breath, bleeding or swollen gums, gnawing hunger pains in the stomach, thirst, frontal headaches radiating to the teeth or gums, and/or mouth sores.

Stomachics are aromatic herbs that promote digestion by circulating and drying dampness.

Summer Heat is an illness often felt in the late summer with symptoms of thirst, aversion to heat, dryness, red face, sweating, irritability, reduced urination, and constipation.

TCM stands for Traditional Chinese Medicine.

Tai Chi or *Tai Ji* is a martial art also used to maintain health. It consists of a series of smooth, fluid movements.

Tao is the way and order of the universe and the philosophy of knowing.

Tonification is to build, nourish, strengthen, or support the Qi, blood, yin, yang, or organs.

Toxins or *Toxic Heat* are pathogens producing extreme fire symptoms of inflammation, infection, cancer, or severe heat disease.

Triple Burner or *Triple Warmer* or *San Jiao* is the collective name for the three body cavities. The upper burner is the heart and lungs, the middle burner is the spleen, stomach, liver, and gallbladder, and the lower burner is the kidney, bladder, and intestines.

Tui Na is a Chinese massage technique using meridians and acupuncture points (see Chapter 1, "Methods of Chinese Medicine").

Wei Qi refers to the defensive energy or immune system.

Wind is a climactic or body condition of obvious or sudden change. Wind invading from outside the body causes sudden and acute conditions like colds, flu, or other infectious diseases. Internal wind causes strokes, twitches, and paralysis.

Yang represents the function of the organs as well as all metabolic activity that generates warmth and circulation.

Yang Deficiency is a lack of yang energy that leads to internal cold and low metabolism. Symptoms include feeling tired, feeling cold, having weak knees or low back and hip pain, and low libido.

Yin represents the structure of the organs and the cooling fluids of the body. This includes blood and bodily fluids that feed, clean, and moisten the organs.

Yin Deficiency is a lack of yin fluids that results in dryness, structural problems, or empty heat.

Zang Fu refers to the twelve organs of the body (see Chapter 3 "Understanding Theories of Chinese Medicine").

Index

Acanthopanax. See wu jia pi
accumulations, 98–99
acne, 72–74
aconite root. *See fu zi*
Aconitum Compound pills. *See fu zi li zhong wan*
acupuncture, 1–2
  how it works, 2
  needle placement, 32–33
  practical suggestions, 23–24
  practiced by Western medical doctors, 11
  sensations felt during, 22–23
acupuncture pointers, 22–23
acupuncturists
  educational requirements and accreditation, 12–14
  "primary care physician" status, 11–12
acute problems, 16–17
addictions, 73–74
adjuvant herbs, 51–52
Agastach pogostemi. See huo xiang
Airborne, 52
alcohol addiction, 73–74
allergies, 75–76
allergy formulas, xanthium-based, 66–68
aloeswood chen xiang, 98
Alzheimer's disease, 76–77
Amomum Nourish Stomach pill. *See xiang sha yang wei wan*
amur cork bark. *See huang bai*
An Tai Wan, 128

Anemarrhena radix. See zhi mu
anemarrhenae asphodeloidis, Radix. See zhi mu
Angelica dahurica. See bai zhi
Angelica sinensis. See dang gui
anger, 36
anxiety, 68–70, 100–101, 131–32
Aquilaria pills, 98
Aquilaria Stomachic pills, 98
arbor vitae seed. *See bai zhi ren*
Arctium lappa. See niu bang zi
arthritis, 16, 77–78
  causes, 78–79
  treatments, 79–80
asthma, 80–82
astragali, Radix. See huang qi
astragalus root. *See huang qi*
astringents, 188–89
Atractylodes radix. See bai zhu
attention-deficit hyperactivity disorder (ADHD), 82–83
aucklandia. *See xiang sha yang wei wan*

ba zhen wan, 57–59
back pain, 83–84
  causes, 84
  herbal treatments, 85
  lower, 84
  upper, 84
bai bu, 134
bai ji tan, 65
bai shao, 55, 58

bai zhi, 58, 60, 67, 68, 138
bai zhi ren, 69
bai zhu, 56, 60, 64, 69, 96–97
balloon flower. *See jie geng*
ban lan gen, 94, 95
ban xia, 64, 170–71
betel nut. *See bing lang*
bi syndrome, 78–80
bing lang, 194
bing pian, 192
Biota semen. See bai zhi ren
bitter melon. *See ku gua*
bitter orange, unripe. *See tao ren*
black cohosh. *See sheng ma*
bleeding
    herbs to stop, 177–79
    products used to stop, 86–87
bleeding disorders, 85–86
blood
    herbs that regulate, 175–76
    herbs to vitalize, 176–77
    Qi and, 29
blood deficiency, 113, 116, 131–32, 150
blood-heat, 110
blood pressure
    herbal treatments to decrease, 124
    herbal treatments to increase, 124–25
    high, 123–25
blood stagnation, 45, 111
blood vessels, patency of, 116
bo he, 56, 60, 138
bodywork, 3
Bojenmi Tea, 151–52
borneol camphor. *See bing pian*
breast cancer, 89
Bright Eyes Rehmannia combination.
        See ming mu di huang
bulrush. *See deng xin cao*
Bupleurum chinense. See chai hu
burdock. *See niu bang zi*
bursitis, 77–78
    causes, 78–79
    treatments, 79–80

California, 11–12
    Proposition 65 warning labels,
        21–22
California Safe Drinking Water and
        Toxic Environment Act, 21–22
Calm Colon, 133
cancer, 87
    causes, 87–88, 145
    disease condition, 87
    treatment, 88–91, 143
cang er zi, 66–68, 168
cang er zi wan, 66–68
Cannabis sativa semen. See huo ma ren
Carthami tinctori flo. See hong hua
cathartics, harsh, 164–65
Certified Acupuncturist (CA), 12
chai hu, 55, 56, 100–101
channel pain, 84
checking cycle, 34
chemotherapy, herbs to treat side
        effects of, 90–91
chen pi, 60, 64, 138, 174–75
chest Qi, constraint of, 106
chien chin chih tai wan, 148
China tung shueh pills, 141
Chinese food, 151
Chinese medicine practitioners. *See*
        traditional Chinese medicine
        (TCM) practitioner(s)
cholesterol, high, 91–92, 121
chronic ailments, 17
chronic fatigue, 112–13
Chrysanthemomi flos. See ju hua
chuan xiong, 58, 67
Cinnamomi ramulus. See gui zhi
cinnamon bark. *See rou gui*
Citri immaturus fructus. See zhi ke
Citri rubrum exocarpum. See chen pi
citrus peel. *See chen pi*
cocklebur fruit. *See cang er zi*
Codonopsis radix. See dang shen
Coicis semen. See yi yi ren

coix lachryma jobi. See yi yi ren
cold, common, 27, 28, 52, 92–93
  prevention, 96–97
  relieving, 95–96
  stopping it early, 93–95
cold (temperature), 127. *See also* hot/
  cold; warming the interior
colon cancer, 89
Concha ostreae. See mu li
constipation, 97–98, 106
cool pungent herbs for releasing the
  exterior, 156–58
Cool the Blood and Expel Wind, 110
cooling blood, herbs for, 110, 158–59.
  See also heat, herbs that clear
Coptidis rhizoma. See huang lian
Cordyceps sinensis. See dong chong xia cao
Cortex cinnamomi cassiae. See rou gui
Cortex phellodendri. See huang bai
cortex radices. *See wu jia pi*
costus root. *See mu xiang*
coughing, 168, 171
Crataegi fructus. See shan za
crested grass. *See dan zhu ye*
curculigo. See xian mao
curculinginis orchiodis, Rhizoma. See
  xian mao
cysts, 98–99

da huang, 97, 163
damp bi syndrome, 46
damp/dry (TCM principle), 32
dampness, 73
  herbs that drain, 165–67
  herbs that dry, 160
  herbs that expel, 167–68
  herbs to transform, 172–73
  yeast and, 146–47
dan dou chi, 54
dan shen, 69
dan zhu ye, 54
dang gui, 51, 58, 66, 98, 175–76
dang shen, 58, 64

deafness, 107
decoctions, 6
  how to drink, 19–20
defensive Qi, 37
deng xin cao, 69
depression, 100–101
desmodium. *See jin qian cao*
diabetes, 101–2
  herbal treatments, 102
  TCM research, 102–3
diagnosis, 9, 10, 15, 16
diarrhea
  cold, 106–7
  herbs for, 106–7
  hot, 106–7
diet recommendations, 151
digestion, slow, 105
digestive problems, 103–4. *See also*
  irritable bowel syndrome
  herbal treatments, 105–7, 151–52
  non-herbal treatments, 104–5
digestive Qi, weak, 105
Diplomate in Acupuncture (Dipl.
  Ac.), 13–14
disease(s). *See also under* treatment,
  case studies
  locating and understanding the
  nature of, 30
Doctor of Oriental Medicine (DOM/
  OMD), 13
dong chong xia cao, 185–86
drug addictions, 73–74
Dryobalanops aromatica. See bing pian

ear ringing, 107
  deficiency, 107–8
  excess, 107
earth element, 33, 34
eating habits, 151
eczema, 108–9
  herbal treatments, 109
Eight Principles, 30–32
Eight Treasures. *See ba zhen wan*

elements. *See* Five Phases
elixirs, how to take, 20
emotions
    excessive, 121
    five, 36–37
energy issues, 112–13. *See also* Qi
epemidii. See xian ling pi
Ephedra sinensis. See ma huang
epilepsy, 113–15
Epimedium sagittatum. See yin yang huo
Er Xiang Wan, 64–66, 136–37
erectile dysfunction, 47–48
Eriobotrya folium. See pi pa ye
esophageal cancer, 89
evodia leaf. *See san cha ku*
excess/deficient (TCM principle), 31
exercise, 120

fang feng. See ledebouriellae sesloidis radix
fatigue, 42–44
fear, 36
feelings, 36–37
fever, 122
fire. *See* heat
Five Phases, 33–36, 40, 42
    correspondences associated with, 34
Five Seed pill. *See* Wu Ren Wan
fleece flower root. *See he shou wu*
Flos lonicera japonic. See jin yin hua
flow, 28–29, 84
flu, 52, 92–93. *See also* cold
fo ti. See he shou wu
Fog Tea, 75
Folium nelumbinis. See he ye
food allergies, 76
food stagnation, herbs relieving, 173–74
Forsythia suspensa fructus. See Lian Qiao
Four Gentlemen. *See si jun zi wan*
foxglove root, Chinese. *See sheng di huang; shu di huang*
Free and Easy. *See hsiao yao san*
Fructus gardenia jasminoidis. See zhi zi
Fructus persica. See tao ren

Fructus schisandrae chinensis. See wu wei zi
Fructus xanthium. See cang er zi
fu, 38
fu ling, 56, 58, 60, 64, 69, 138, 165–66
fu zheng gu ben, 87, 88, 143
fu zi, 62
fu zi li zhong wan, 139

gambir vine. *See gou teng*
gan cao, 54, 56, 58, 70, 124
Gan Lu Qing Re Pian, 139
gan mao ling, 94–95
Ganoderma lucida. See ling zhi
Gardenia semen. See zhi zi
gastric reflux diseases (GRD), 105, 137. *See also* digestive problems
Gastrodia rhiz. See tian ma
Gate of Life, 39
ge gen, 60, 67, 68, 75, 95, 138–39, 156–57
ge hua, 75, 156–58
generating cycle, 34
ginger. *See sheng jiang*
ginseng. *See ren shen*
ginseng, American. *See xi yang shen*
ginseng, Siberian. *See wu jia pi*
Glycyrrhiza uranelsis radix. See gan cao
goiter, 145
gold coin herb. *See jin qian cao*
Golden Book pills, 142–43. *See also gui fu di huang; jin gui di huang wan*
golden thread. *See huang lian*
Good Sleep and Worry Free Pill, 68–70
gou teng, 192–93
granules, 6, 20–21
Grave's disease, 145
grief, 36
gu ya, 60, 138
gui fu di huang, 61, 62. *See also* Golden Book pills

gui zhi, 97
Gypsum fibrosum. See shi gao

hai zao, 169
hair, prematurely gray, 115–17
hair loss, 116–17
hairy holly root. *See mao tung ching*
hangover, 119
hare's ear root. *See chai hu*
Hashimoto's complex, 145
hawthorn berry. *See shan za*
he huan pi, 101
he shou wu, 116–17
he ye, 162
headaches, 117–19
health care system, Chinese medicine
    in, 26–27
health insurance coverage, 25–26
heart
    disharmony between kidneys and,
        132
    herbs that nourish, 189–90
heart attack, 121
heart blood deficiency, 131–32. *See
    also* blood deficiency
heart health, 119–21
heart of poria. *See fu ling*
heartburn, 105. *See also* digestive
    problems
heat, 72–73, 81–82, 110, 111, 127. *See
    also* hot/cold
    congested, 84
    deficiency, 132
    herbs that clear, 158–62. *See also*
        cooling blood
    liver, 81
    menopause and, 135
heat treatment. *See* moxibustion
Heavenly Emperor Strengthen Heart
    Pill. *See tian huang bu xin wan*
hemorrhoids, 122–23
hepatitis, 121–22
herb of the cross. *See ma pien tsao*

*Herba agastaches seu pogostemi. See huo
    xiang*
Herba artemisae. See qing hao
Herba ephedra. See ma huang
Herba verbenae. See ma pien tsao
herbal formulas. *See also* herbs, value
    of combining
    famous, 52. *See also specific formulas*
    how they are created, 51–52
herbal pills
    how to take, 18–19
    what to take with, 19
herbal pointers, 17–18
herbal therapy, 5–7
herbs, 154
    functions, 51–52
    purity, 72
    that drain downward, 162–65
    that release exterior conditions,
        155–58
    that strengthen, 180. *See also*
        tonifying herbs
    value of combining, 50–51
    ways of preparing and ingesting,
        5–7
herpes simplex, 153
herpes zoster, 153
hoelin mushroom. *See fu ling*
honeysuckle. *See jin yin hua*
honeysuckle flowers. *See jin yin hua*
hong hua, 177–78
hormones, 135–36
horny goat weed. *See yin yang huo*
hot/cold (TCM principle), 31. *See also*
    heat
hot flashes, 134–37
hou po, 60, 138
hsiao yao san, 54–57
huang bai, 61, 62, 65
huang jing cao, 94
huang lian, 160
huang qi (astragalus), 96, 125, 180–81
    other herbs combined with, 181

hunger, 151
huo ma ren, 164
huo xiang, 60, 67, 68, 138, 172–73
Huperzia serotta, 77
hyperactivity, 82–83
hyperthyroid, 145, 146
hypothyroid, 145

illicis pubescentis, Radix. See mao tung ching
immunity, 125
    bolstering, 96–97, 125
in vitro fertilization (IVF), 126–28
indigo. *See ban lan gen*
infertility, 125–26
    deficiency pattern, 126
    heat or cold pattern, 127
    stagnation pattern, 126–27
injury, 129–31
    third-stage, 79, 130–31
inside/outside (TCM principle), 31
insomnia, 42–44, 68–70, 131–32
irritable bowel syndrome (IBS), 132–33
isatidis, Radix. See ban lan gen
isatis root. *See ban lan gen*

Jade Shield/Jade Windscreen, 96
jaundice, 122
jia wei xiao yao wan, 55
jiao gu lan, 92
jie geng, 53
jin bu huan, 141
jin gui di huang wan, 85
jin gui shen qi wan, 48, 49, 61
jin qian cao, 166–67
jin yin hua, 53, 94, 161
jing jie, 53, 54
Job's tears. *See yi yi ren*
joint pain, 77–78
    causes, 78–79
    treatments, 79–80
joy, 36
ju hua, 60, 67, 68, 94, 138

jujube seed, sour. *See suan zao ren*

Kai Kit Prostate Gland pill, 142
kidney Qi deficiency, 45, 48–49, 81, 82, 113, 143–44
kidneys, 43
    disharmony between heart and, 132
ko ning wan, 59–60. *See also* Stomach Curing pills
ku gua, 102
ku shen, 134
kudzu flower. *See ge hua*
kudzu root. *See ge gen*

laxatives, moist, 163–64
leaven, medicated. *See shen qu*
ledebouriellae sesloidis radix, 97
Lian Qiao, 53
lice, 133–34
licorice root, Chinese. *See gan cao*
Lignum aquilaria. See aloeswood chen xiang
Liguistici wallichi. See chuan xiong
Ligustri lucidi fructus. See nu zhen zi
ling zhi, 184–85
Liquidambar fructus. See lu lu tong
Liquidambar styraciflua, 67
listening (examination), 9
liu huang, 195
liu jun zi wan, 63–64
liu wei, 62
liu wei di huang, 61–63
liver, 42–43, 122
    hot, 105
    not smoothing Qi, 79
liver blood deficiency, 150
liver cancer, 90
liver heat, 81
liver yin deficiency, 79
long gu muli xiao yao wan, 55
Lonicera flos. See jin yin hua
looking (examination), 9
Lophatheri gracilis. See dan zhu ye

loquat leaf. *See pi pa ye*
lotus leaf. *See he ye*
lovage root. *See chuan xiong*
lu lu tong, 67, 68
lung cancer, 89–90
lung Qi deficiency, 81, 82
lung tan xie gan wan, 148
lysimachia. *See jin qian cao*

ma huang, 124, 155–56
ma pien tsao, 95
Magnolia cortex. See hou po
Magnolia flos. See xin ye hua
mai men dong, 98
Man's Treasure formulas. *See nan bao*
mao tung ching, 95
marijuana seeds. *See huo ma ren*
Massa fermentata. See shen qu
massage, 3
Medical Acupuncturists, 11
Medical Doctor in China (MD
        China), 13
medical history, 16
medications, 15
medicines
    different diseases requiring the
        same, 45–47
    same disease requiring different,
        45–47
Medula junci. See deng xin cao
memory, 83
menopause, 134–37
    yin deficiencies and, 113
Mentha folium. See bo he
Menthe herba. See bo he
meridians, 32–33
messenger herbs, 52
metal element, 33, 34
mi huan jun, 114–15
milk-vetch root. *See huang qi*
milk wort, Siberian. *See zhi mu*
milled powders, 6, 20
ming men. *See* Gate of Life

ming mu di huang, 61
mint leaf. *See bo he*
miscarriage
    causes and herbal treatments,
        128–29
Moisten Intestines pill. *See run chang
    wan*
Momordica charantia. See ku gua
More Energy from Less Food
        Powder, 152
morinda officianalis, Radix. See bai ji tan
Morinda root. *See bai ji tan*
morning glory seeds. *See qian niu zi*
morning sickness, 137. *See also* nausea
movement, 28–29
    and health, 4
moxibustion, 2–3
mu li, 66, 190–91
mu xiang, 59, 138

nan bao, 144
National Committee for the
        Certification of Acupuncture
        and Oriental Medicine
        (NCCAOM), 12–14
nausea, 137–39
New Mexico, 11–12
nicotine addiction, 73–74
niu bang zi, 54
niu pi xuan er hao fang, 111
niu pi xuan hao fang, 110
No More Lice Herbal Shock, 134
notoginseng. *See tienchi*
notopterygi. *See qiang huo*
*notopterygium incisium, Radix. See
    qiang huo*
*notopterygium incisium, Rhizome. See
    qiang huo*
nu zhen zi, 96

OMD (Doctor of Oriental
        Medicine), 13
ophiopogon tuber. *See mai men dong*

organ systems, 34, 35, 45
organic herbs, 184
organs, twelve, 37–39
orifices, aromatic herbs that open,
       191–92
Oryzae germinantus. See gu ya
ovarian cancer, 89
overeating, 105
oyster shell. *See mu li*

Paeonia. See bai shao
pain, 122, 129–31
       causes, 140
       disease condition, 139
       flow and, 32
       herbal treatment, 140
       non-herbal treatments, 140
pain medicines, general, 141
*panacis quinquefolii, Radix. See xi yang
       shen*
panax ginseng, Radix. See ren shen
Panax ginseng rx. See ren shen
Panax quinquefolius. See xi yang shen
parasites
       herbs that expel, 193–94
patchouli. *See huo xiang*
patients
       what practitioners expect from,
              14–16
pe min kan wan, 66–68
Peaceful Fetus pill. *See An Tai Wan*
Peach Kernel pill. *See run chang wan*
peach seed kernel. *See tao ren*
Peonia lactiflora. See bai shao
peppermint. *See bo he*
Pericarpium citri reticulatae. See chen pi
Persica semen. See tao ren
Pharbitides semen. See qian niu zi
phlegm
       cold, 169–71
       herbs that transform, 168–71
       hot, 169
physicians, Western, 24

pi pa ye, 171
Pinellia ternata. See ban xia
Platycodi grandiflori radix. See jie geng
Po Chai pills. *See ko ning wan*;
       Stomach Curing pills
Polygoni multiflori. See he shou wu
Poria cocos sclerotum. See fu ling
powders, milled, 6
pregnancy, 128. *See also* morning
       sickness
preperatum, Rhizoma. See ban xia
principal herbs, 51
privet fruit. *See nu zhen zi*
prostate cancer, 143
prostate conditions, 141–43
prostate specific antigen (PSA) levels,
       143
prostatitis
       acute, 142
       deficiency type, 142
pseudoginseng. *See tienchi*
psoriasis, 108–10
       caused by blood-heat and stasis, 110
       caused by flaming of heat-evil
              combined with wind, 110
       caused by toxic-heat and blood-
              stasis, 111
       external treatments, 111
Pueraria flos. See ge hua
Pueraria radix. See ge gen
pulse, quality/type of, 10
purgatives, 163

Qi, 3, 22–23, 28–29, 36–37. *See also
       specific topics*
       excess, 84
       herbs that regulate, 174–75
       stagnation, 45–46, 116. *See also*
              stagnation
       stuck, 84
       weak, 84
qi gong, 4
qi ye lian, 141

qian niu zi, 164–65
qiang huo, 96
qing hao, 95–96
Quisqualis indica fructus. See bing lang

radiation, herbs to treat side effects of, 90–91
Rambling Powder. See hsiao yao san
Ramulus uncaria cum uncis. See gou teng
reflux, 105. See also digestive problems
Rehmannia Eight Combination. See zhi bai di huang
Rehmannia glutinosa radix. See sheng di huang; shu di huang
Rehmannia radix. See sheng di huang
Rehmannia Six Combination. See liu wei di huang
rei, Rhizoma. See da huang
reishi/rei shi mushroom. See ling zhi
Relaxed Wanderer. See hsiao yao san
ren shen (ginseng), 69, 181–84
and blood pressure, 124
extracts, 183
organic, 184
preparation, 184
price, 183
restlessness, 131–32
Rhei rhizoma. See da huang
Rhizoma rei. See da huang
Rhubarb radix. See da huang
rhubarb rhizome, Chinese. See da huang
rice sprout. See gu ya
rou gui, 62, 179–80
Ruin Your Appetite Powder, 152
run chang wan, 97, 98

sadness, 36
safflower. See hong hua
sage root, Chinese. See dan shen
Salvia radix. See dan shen
san cha ku, 94
san qi. See tienchi
Sargassi herba. See hai zao

Saussureae radix. See mu xiang
Schefflera Root Relieve Pain. See qi ye lian
Schisandra fructus. See wu wei zi
Schizonepeta tenuifolia. See jing jie
seaweed. See hai zao
seizures, 113–15
yang/closed, 115
yin/open, 114–15
Sexoton pills. See jin gui shen qi wan
sexual problems, 143–144
shan za, 91–92, 173–74
shen, 68, 120
disturbed, 131
shen qu, 138
sheng di huang, 98, 159
sheng jiang, 56
sheng ma, 136
shi gao, 96
Shi San Tai Pao Wan, 128
shiatsu, 3
shu di huang, 58, 61
si jun zi wan, 63–64
side effects, 51. See also adjuvant herbs
siler. See ledebouriellae sesloidis radix
sinus pills, 66–68
Six Gentlemen. See liu jun zi wan
skin diseases, inflammatory, 108
smelling and tasting (examination), 9
smoking. See nicotine addiction
Sojae praeparatum semen. See dan dou chi
sour date seed. See suan zao ren
soy bean, fermented. See dan dou chi
spirit, herbs that settle, 189–91
spleen Qi deficiency, 63, 81, 112–13
stagnation, 88, 126–27
blood, 45, 111
food, 173–74
Qi, 45–46, 116
stomach cancer, 89
Stomach Curing pills, 137–39. See also ko ning wan
stress, 54–56

stroke, 121
suan zao ren, 69, 190
sulphur. *See liu huang*
summer heat, herbs that relieve,
    161–62
supporting herbs, 51
Sweet Dew Clear Heat tablet. *See*
    Gan Lu Qing Re Pian
swelling, 98–99
Szechuan lovage root. *See chuan xiong*

tai chi, 5
tangerine peel, aged. *See chen pi*
tangkuei/tang gui root. *See dang gui*
tao ren, 98
tea, steeped, 7
tendonitis, 45–47, 77–78
    causes, 78–79
    treatments, 79–80
Thirteen Weeks Great Protecting pill.
    See Shi San Tai Pao Wan
thyroid, 48
thyroid problems, 144–46
tian huang bu xin wan, 61
tian ma, 60, 114–15, 138
tian ma mi huan, 114–15
tian qi. *See tienchi*
tienchi, 86, 178–79
tinctures, how to take, 20
tinnitus. *See ear ringing*
tong bian wan, 98
tonifying herbs, 180
tonifying Qi, herbs for, 180–85
tonifying yang, herbs for, 185–87
tonifying yin, herbs for, 187–88
topical application, herbs for, 195
touching (examination), 10
toxins, herbs for cleaning, 161
traditional Chinese medicine (TCM)
    practitioner(s)
    accreditation and kinds of, 11–14
    applying the theories of, 40
    first visit with, 8

training, 11
    vs. Western doctors, 8
    what patients expect from, 9–10
trauma, 129–31
Treasure from the Golden Cabinet.
    See gui fu di huang
treatment
    case studies, 41–44
    same disease, different
        medicines, 45–47
    same medicine, different
        diseases, 47–49
    cost, 24–26
    length, 16–17
treatment sessions, number of, 16
tremors, herbs that stop, 192–93
tui na, 3
tumors, 98–99, 146. *See also* cancer
Two Immortals pill. *See Er Xiang Wan*
types, five, 35

urination, frequent, 49

vaginal discharge, 148
vaginal dryness, 149
vaginal itching, 148, 149
vaginal yeast infections, 146–49
vervain. *See ma pien tsao*
viral disease, 152. *See also* cold
    prolonged, 113
vitex herb. *See huang jing cao*
vomiting, 137–39

warm pungent herbs for releasing
    the exterior, 155–56
warming the interior. *See also* cold
    (temperature)
    herbs for, 179–80
warts, 149–50
wei qi, vacuity of, 46
weight gain, weight loss, and diets,
    150–52
wheezing, 171

wind
   herbs that expel, 167–68
   herbs that extinguish interior,
      191–92
woad root. *See ban lan gen*
Women's Precious Pill. *See ba zhen wan*
wood element, 33, 34
wormwood plant. *See qing hao*
wu jia pi, 167
Wu Ren Wan, 98
wu wei zi, 69, 188–89
wu xing, 33–35

xanthium-based allergy formulas,
   66–68
Xanthium fructus. See cang er zi
xi yang shen, 103, 187–88
xian ling pi, 65
xian mao, 65
xiang sha yang wei wan, 139
xiao yao san. See hsiao yao san
xiao yao wan, 67
xin ye hua, 67, 68

ya dan zi, 149
yeast infections, vaginal, 146–49
yi yi ren, 60, 138
yin and yang, 43
   balance, harmony, and change,
      29–30, 43
   examples, 30
   functions, 38–39
   organs associated with, 38
yin chiao chieh tu pien, 52–54, 93–94
yin yang huo, 65, 186–87
yudai wan, 147
yunnan paiyao/yunnan baiyao, 86–87

zai zao wan, 115
zhang, 38
zhi bai di huang, 61, 62
zhi gan cao, 58, 64
zhi ke, 98

zhi mu, 61, 62, 65, 69, 136
zhi zi, 69, 158–59
Zinzeberis. See sheng jiang
Zizyphus semen. See suan zao ren
zong gan ling, 95–96